C000109739

# The Psychodynamics of Addiction

© 2002 Whurr Publishers

First published 2002 by
Whurr Publishers Ltd
19b Compton Terrace, London N1 2UN, England, and
325 Chestnut Street, Philadelphia PA 19106, USA

Reprinted 2003

All rights reserved. No part of this publication may be
reproduced, stored in a retrieval system, or transmitted in
any form or by any means, electronic, mechanical, photo-
copying, recording or otherwise, without the prior
permission of Whurr Publishers Limited.

This publication is sold subject to the conditions that it
shall not, by way of trade or otherwise, be lent, resold,
hired out, or otherwise circulated without the Publisher's
prior consent, in any form or binding or cover other than
that in which it was published, and without a similar
condition being imposed upon any subsequent purchaser.

**British Library Cataloguing in Publication Date**
A catalogue record for this book is available from the
British Library.

ISBN 1 86156 335 3

Printed and bound in the UK by Athenaeum Press Ltd,
Gateshead, Tyne & Wear

# Contents

# Contributors

**Robert Cohen** Consultant Addiction Psychiatrist, DDU, Homerton Hospital, London

**Robert Hale** Consultant Psychiatrist and Psychotherapist, Medical Director, Portman Clinic, London

**Arthur Hyatt Williams** Retired Consultant Psychiatrist and Psychoanalyst, London

**Francis Keaney** Clinical Tutor at the Institute of Psychiatry and Honorary Senior Registrar, South London and Maudsley Trust

**MaryAnn Lysaght** Psychotherapist, Cassel Hospital, London

**James Mosse** Psychotherapist, Developmental Disabilities Division, St Andrew's Hospital, Northampton

**Anne Read** Consultant Psychiatrist, Plymouth Community Drug Service

**Bill Reading** Psychotherapist, Manager and Nurse Specialist, Mount Zeehan Hospital, Canterbury, Kent

**Luis Rodríguez de la Sierra** Psychiatrist and Psychoanalyst, Private Practice, London

**Shamil Wanigaratne** Consultant Clinical Psychologist, South London and Maudsley Trust and Honorary Senior Lecturer, Institute of Psychiatry

**Martin Weegmann** Consultant Clinical Psychologist and Group Analyst, Gatehouse Drug Service, Southall, Middlesex

# Foreword

PROFESSOR EDWARD KHANTZIAN

Martin Weegmann and Robert Cohen, the editors of *The Psychodynamics of Addiction*, have compiled a genre of work of which there have been far too few. Addiction is the single most pervasive public and mental health problem of our time. The breadth and scope of the problem seems to leave programmes and practitioners pressed to offer acute management and quick solutions, with little time or inclination to explore and address, at a deeper psychological level, the more complex determinants of addictive behaviour. This book provides rich clinical and theoretical material that will stimulate students and clinicians better to appreciate core issues of suffering and dysregulation ('container and contained') that are central to addictive vulnerability. From the outset the editors and authors deal with the complexities of addictive suffering. They set the stage by introducing three psychoanalytic paradigms to explore the world of the addicted person. Three views are adopted – Bion's emphasis on self-containment, Bowlby's perspective on the process of attachment and Kohut's probing of human narcissistic vulnerability – and provide an ample framework to face one of the most central problems of addictions, 'the capacity to face mental pain'.

In my experience two crucial problems are at the heart of addictive disorders: (1) human psychological suffering and (2) the inability to control one's life. In the former instance, human issues of experiencing emotions (or affects) are in the extreme: patients' feelings are overwhelming and unbearable or they are absent and confusing. In the latter cases, patients alternate between losing control of their behaviours and substances, and then, often at the same time, they exert multiple and varied attempts to gain and maintain control. These polarities have ultimately led me to adopt a perspective of addictions as a self-regulation disorder. I have repeatedly emphasised the importance of a disordered sense of self and related difficulties in maintaining self-esteem. Not surprisingly, one consequence of a disordered sense of self is a disordered capacity to relate to others. These are important and contributory factors to addictive vulnerability. Important as these factors are in contributing to addictions, I have concluded that disturbances in regulating affects and behaviours malignantly combine and are essential in the development of addictive disorders.

Weegmann, Cohen and associates provide extensive evidence in their collective efforts to support a perspective of substance use and misuse as a self-regulation disorder involving deficits in regulating self-esteem, relationships, affect and behaviours (particularly self-care). In the first chapter Hyatt Williams draws on Bion's concept of the container and the contained and explores how people with infantile feelings of emptiness or the distress of separation, often played out in the transference, resort to drugs to contain feelings that are otherwise uncontainable. Chronically doing so further lessens a person's capacity to manage and regulate his or her emotions. In my own work I have used the term 'disuse atrophy' to characterise this process. That is, albeit adaptive when drugs are used initially, ultimately chronic dependence on addictive drugs undermines an already diminished capacity to endure or tolerate psychic pain. This is the sorrowful and illusory nature of addictive disorders; drugs are compelling because they initially work, but ultimately because of physical tolerance and evolving diminished psychological capacities, the attempts at self-correction tragically fail. Little wonder, as Hyatt Williams (and Rado, whom he cites) indicates, that suicide often becomes a fatal alternative. Hyatt Williams concludes by encouraging treating clinicians to address 'the progressive loss of containment' as a critical focus of our therapeutic efforts.

Bill Reading in his chapter on attachment theory, draws on the work of Bowlby and provides us with another pivotal area upon which therapists can focus. Namely, as in other models of psychotherapy, attachment theory can help clinicians 'enhance the patient's ability to locate his or her symptoms in an interpersonal context'. McLellan and associates have empirically demonstrated this by exploring how 'core conflictual relationship themes' (CCRT) play themselves out in the treatment relationship and provide the therapist and patient a basis for understanding how these themes precipitate and maintain a dependence on substances. We have similarly described how self-regulation disturbances, especially interpersonal ones, play themselves in the group interactions in modified group therapy (Khantzian et al 1990) and provide opportunities to enhance self-observation and modify behaviours that predispose to and make more likely a reliance on addictive substances.

The authors in this volume appreciate well why simply identifying triggers for relapse and related cognitive behavioural treatments alone are not sufficient to prevent use and reversion to addictive behaviours. They repeatedly and astutely provide sophisticated underpinning for Rado's assertion that it is not the drug but the impulse to use it. It is only through appreciating the deeper psychodynamic layers of vulnerabilities and developmental deficits, which are supplied in this book, that we can appreciate why addictive drugs are so compelling. Weegmann's chapter on the vulnerable self provides an important appreciation, based on Kohut's work, of how fundamental disruptions in self-organisations cause individuals to resort to substances to compensate for deficits in self-structures. When these structures are absent, individuals are prone to addiction because they cannot achieve or maintain inner coherence, they cannot comfort themselves, and they are unable to soothe themselves or assure their self-care. Thus, such individuals are chronically uncomfortable from within and more often in harm's way when faced with external danger, including and in particular the self-harm of addictive drug use.

With this foundation of understanding, Weegmann and his associates instruct and guide the reader through the challenges of appreciating the psychodynamics of engaging patients and assessing them in treatment. They emphasise the subtleties of patient encounters, helping the clinicians to be patient and empathic, to be ready for denial and ambivalence, to anticipate and expect resistance and overt hostility but ultimately to trust that the clinician and patient can gradually build a relationship that enables understanding and a means to relinquish the patient's maladaptive/immature patterns and their attachment to their drug-of-choice. These psychodynamic precepts are consistently honoured and sustained in the chapters on individual therapy by Read and group psychotherapy by Mosse and Lysaght and imaginatively integrated in a chapter by Wanigaratne and Keaney on relapse-prevention groups. The editors provide a bonus with relevant and enlightening chapters on supervision and the vicissitudes of countertransference in chapters by Hale and Rodríguez de la Sierra respectively. The final chapter on growing up with addiction by Weegmann takes us beyond superficial aphorisms of what it is like and again upholds the main thrust and commitment of this book, namely to explore in depth the inner workings and psychological structures of an addictive adaptation, in this case how it works in addicted families.

I applaud Martin Weegmann and Robert Cohen in undertaking the challenge of compiling this psychodynamic treatise on the addictions. They have carefully designed a focus and assembled a team of knowledgeable and sophisticated clinicians who uphold the rigour and challenges of providing an in-depth exploration of human psychological problems, in this case the problem of addictive disorders. They truly appreciate the nature of this special adaptation which for so many on the surface seems simply to be a self-destructive maladaptation. The sophisticated understanding and time-honoured clinical traditions of psychodynamic psychiatry combine with compassion and empathy in *The Psychodynamics of Addiction* to bring alive and make more manageable one of the most daunting maladies of our time: addictive vulnerability and suffering.

# Preface

Amongst healthcare professionals, people who have problems with alcohol or drug use are not popular. Views such as 'it's a self-inflicted condition', 'they are so difficult to treat' or 'I don't like them' are common.

Such views reflect prejudice. There is a wealth of evidence nowadays that shows that addiction is a biopsychosocial disorder that is rightly included as a group of diseases by the World Health Organisation in the *International Classification of Diseases* (tenth edition, categories F10–19). In other words, we are starting to get some understanding of the different biological, psychological and social processes that lead to a significant number of the population using psychoactive drugs and coming to physical, psychological and social harm as a result. The picture that we have shows that addiction is a complex, multifaceted disorder. Criticising an addict is no different from criticising someone because they are poor or because they are bleeding from a stomach ulcer (which may have been caused by years of stress).

It is not easy to know how to treat people who show a range of difficult behaviours, but, as with all areas within psychological disturbance and psychiatry, we should try to understand these behaviours, because, if we do, we may be able to handle them effectively for the benefit of the addict, those closest to him or her and those trying to assist him or her, both professionally or otherwise.

For example, people who are intoxicated will often turn up at accident and emergency departments of local hospitals. There they may meet an inexperienced nurse or doctor, who tells them off in a most officious way for 'doing it to themselves'. Sometimes, the patient does not take kindly to this and assaults the staff member verbally or, occasionally, physically. The patient is removed from the hospital, any underlying medical condition remains untreated. The nurse or doctor is relieved, but disgusted at having to have dealt with another difficult drunk.

But, if we consider what has really happened, we can gain an understanding of what went wrong and why the outcome was unsatisfactory for both parties.

All human beings need to feel that they are decent people. Our own opinion of ourselves is very important: if we think that we are not good enough – because of lack of money, girlfriend/boyfriend, academic or sporting achievement, good looks, status in society, or whatever other reason – we feel unhappy and depressed. Those who have experience of addicts, treating them directly or studying them psychologically, know that self-esteem amongst addicts, whatever their drug, is low. As a rule, addicts don't think much of themselves.

Telling someone off is a very good way of lowering their self-esteem. And when our self-esteem is attacked, we are often tempted to retaliate.

So we have all the ingredients for what happens in casualty departments all around the world, every day. An addict with low self-esteem attends a casualty department where he or she is told off by a person in authority. With already damaged self-esteem being attacked further, the verbally or physically aggressive behaviour of the addict is entirely understandable

This behaviour does not become acceptable because we understand it. But many more experienced nurses and doctors in those same casualty departments do use this understanding to prevent the violent incidents in the first place. They speak respectfully, but realistically, to patients. Like their more inexperienced colleagues, they may have nothing to offer the addict at the time they come to the casualty department, but, by understanding something of the nature of addiction, they prevent the situation escalating to becoming unpleasant for all concerned.

Note that, so far, we have not mentioned alcohol or drugs as a reason for the patient's behaviour. There is no evidence at present to suggest that the act of taking alcohol or another drug directly causes the person to have chronic low self-esteem. Attack the self-esteem of a non-addict hard enough in the casualty department and you can provoke the same response (though it is true that the self-control of an individual is impaired when intoxicated).

But this is an example of how knowledge of some of the psychological aspects of addiction can be used for the benefit of the patient or their family and friends, and for healthcare staff.

Much has been written about some of the cognitive-behavioural aspects of the psychology of addiction. These are the conscious thoughts, beliefs and habits that addicts have that lead to continuing drug use. It can be very helpful to look in cognitive-behavioural therapy at the belief systems of the patient and their automatic responses to a given situation to help the patient to try to modify them for the patient's benefit.

But little has been written about the subconscious processes that occur all the time. The treatment of addiction has rightly focused on alcohol- or drug-taking behaviour and the conscious steps that a therapist can use to guide a patient consciously towards giving up drug use.[1] However, for those patients who do not make progress towards a comfortable lifestyle, a great deal can be learned from considering those unconscious processes, or psychodynamics.

This book aims to take a step in filling this gap.

The experts who have contributed to it have all noted in their own clinical practice how psychodynamics can be discerned in the ways people become addicted to drugs, how they behave when they come for treatment and the changes they make when they get towards recovery. We hope that we can help the reader who comes into contact with addicted patients as a therapist at any level to become more aware of these subconscious processes and use this knowledge for the benefit of his or her patients.

Knowledge in psychotherapy has arisen over a long period of time from the observation of myriad therapists of the thoughts and behaviours of individuals whom they have treated. For this reason, the first section of this book places the psychodynamics of addiction within a historical context before moving on to direct clinical illustrations of these ideas.

Current views on patient confidentiality require that no patient should have identifiable details about themselves disclosed to any other person without their express consent. For this reason, all contributors have assured us that any clinical 'case' described is in fact a composite manufactured from the numerous patients they have treated. All personal details used towards a composite have been changed. Thus, if a reader thinks that they can recognise a patient from any of the clinical 'cases', he or she may be reassured that this is not so.

We hope, therefore, that the reader who is less familiar with the psychodynamic aspects of addiction can gain a useful introduction to the subject. We are also sure that the quality and experience of our contributors are such that even a most experienced practitioner in the field will gain something from reading this book.

We would like to take the opportunity to thank those who have assisted us in bringing this project to completion, in particular, Bill Reading and

---

[1] For a clinician, abstinence must be the ultimate goal. This is not for moral reasons, but because, if the patient is showing serious psychological distress by his or her use of alcohol or other drugs, the only full treatment is to help the patient get past that distress. The addict only shows that the distress has eased by reducing his or her use of alcohol or drugs. But the process can take a long time, and it is also appropriate to help the patient avoid coming to an untimely end before reaching the stage of recovery because of one of the known complications with 'harm reduction' measures.

Jason Maratos and colleagues from the Gatehouse Community alcohol and drug teams, Ealing. We would also like to thank Professor Edward Khantzian, a renowned figure in the field of addiction psychotherapy, for doing us the honour of providing the foreword to this book. Shamil Wanigaratne and Francis Keaney would like to acknowledge the assistance of Jessica Kirker and Fiona McGruer.

It has been a privilege to have had the contributions of so many eminent writers and, as editors, we have both enjoyed and benefited from their submissions for this book. We hope and trust that you will do so too.

April 2002

# Part 1
# A review of different schools

# CHAPTER 1

# Container and contained: the school of Bion

## ARTHUR HYATT WILLIAMS

The psychoanalytic work of Bion did not make an explicit study of the psychology of addiction. In a posthumous publication (1992), which contained entries from his diaries, there are just one and a half pages of notes on drug-taking. These begin with the following four statements.

- Drugs are substitutes employed by those who cannot wait.
- The substitute is that which cannot satisfy without destroying the capacity for discriminating the real from the false.
- Whatever is falsely employed as a substitute for the 'real' is transformed thereby into a poison for the mind.
- The substitute of that which is peripheral to action instead of central must cause imbalance.

Bion originated elsewhere a number of psychoanalytic concepts that have a bearing on drug-taking, perhaps the most notable of which is the concept of container and contained. Psychic states and feelings, like other phenomena, have to be contained in order to be rendered manageable and meaningful. For this, some sort of container or containing function is required. Psychically speaking, that which is uncontainable worsens the subject's ability to keep a situation in the mind. Relief is afforded by communication, including in psychoanalysis or psychoanalytic psychotherapy, or it may be achieved through artificial means. An uncontainable situation in the external world is usually something that is consciously feared, hated or unwisely loved. Those who seek relief from such situations through the use of drugs tend to develop a powerful love–hate relationship with the drug of choice. It is not unheard of, for example, for a patient in the hate phase of his or her addiction to throw his or her precious drugs into the lavatory bowl and flush them away, only to

3

become desperate at the loss minutes later and seek more supplies either by prescription or from a dealer. In my own professional work, I have had my signature forged on an NHS prescription form in this way.

The rationalised excuse given by the addict for their addiction is that they fear something or someone in the external world and that taking drugs mitigates the pain. Sometimes a cyclothymic person on a high may use the drug to allay the state of precarious euphoria: this represents a slap-happy rush to action in pursuit of an ill-prepared and unearned state of mental peace. Although this irresponsible attitude is dangerous, it is less problematic to treat than its opposite, namely when the unconscious/conscious intention is to 'cease upon the midnight with no pain'. This intention tends to be suicidal, either by direct and determined self-killing or by chance, for example causing an accident either through the use of drugs or perhaps a traffic violation or through illness, which can include a range of options including AIDS. The illness then acts like an execution warrant and a dice with death takes place.

## How people become addicted

People who become addicted to drugs do so by selection, by accident or by having experienced a psychically or physically painful illness for which a painkiller has been prescribed. This latter category becomes enslaved by the experience of relief afforded by the drug. I had personal experience of treating a patient from this category; he was a doctor who, as a young university student, developed a painful tonsillitis and was given morphia when the pain was unresponsive to minor drugs. When he qualified in medicine several years later he gained access to various kinds of medicines and drugs, and resorted to his old friend morphia by taking small doses. This was the beginning of his addiction. As he gradually became dependent upon the drug, he began to give himself morphia for pain other than that of the body. The dosage he prescribed himself increased as he became 'tolerant' of the drug. Eventually, he could no longer control the amount he took and became utterly dependent for his continued existence on the drug.

The kind of addiction I have described is pathological and dangerous, but drug-taking, even as a daily habit, has been prevalent in some parts of the world for a very long time. In India, for example, some families have used opium for many generations. A member of such a family described for me once how four generations of their family had used opium and that an acceptable balance was maintained unless or until supplies of the drug became restricted. Provided adequate supplies were maintained, the habit could be managed. This type of culturally syntonic drug-taking needs to be distinguished from that which one finds in opium-taking in the West today. This latter category usually exhibits far more profound character problems.

### Psychoanalysts and drug takers

Psychoanalysts have been interested in drug-taking for many decades: in the 1930s a number of analysts, including Simmel, Rado and Glover, discussed the problem. There was general agreement that:

• The psychic use to which the drug is put is more important than the drug itself.
• The underlying cyclothymic personality of the user is significant, but it is generally agreed that it is not quite like manic-depressive illness. However, certain similarities between the drug addict and the manic-depressive person have been noted, although there are also many differences.
• The struggle between life and death instincts was tilted towards death, but in the main the conflict remained open yet unresolved.

In 1960 Herbert Rosenfeld produced a paper on drug addiction and stated that the addict cannot be successfully psychoanalysed without the analytic work reaching back to an earlier phase of life during which there occurred a polarisation between what is felt to be 'good' and what is felt to be 'bad'. In other words, there occurred a wide separation of the present, gratifying breast (or its substitute) from the absent, frustrating and depriving breast. This polarisation increases with the severity of the addictive illness, and, in the most ill addicts, the state of wide polarity of attitude can resemble an oscillation between deification and demonisation.

Such excessive splitting takes place very early in life, far earlier than the negotiation of what Melanie Klein (1946) refers to as the depressive position (or stage of concern for others) and, as a result, the negotiation of that developmental hurdle becomes much more difficult. Their relatively poor development leads addicts to experience fantasies that, as with criminals, tend to be cruel, destructive and violent. A consequence of these volatile states can be that treatment can seem to be almost, but not quite, insuperably difficult. Rosenfeld (1960) states that each step in the attempted reintegration of the ego of the drug addict is followed by an increase in acting out which risks a violent relapse into a more primitive state of mind (as Klein would have it, the paranoid-schizoid position). Sometimes, the scale of the projective identification involved in these negative therapeutic reactions can lead to a premature ending of the treatment.

*Case example*

Let us return to my doctor patient who became addicted to morphia. He was treated by me for many years, and the treatment was held up on numerous occasions and in many different ways, for reasons which seemed to be united in an underlying attitude: 'I am not going to give up my drug for you or anyone else'. Dependence on the drug was more important to him than dependence on any human being. His falsification of reality was often expressed by his loudly stated belief and accusation that I was addicted to morphia just as he was. He acted out this omniscient, incorrect theory by creating prescriptions for opiates and forging them using a fairly good imitation of my signature. I analysed this behaviour with him, and this produced a sad and reproachful gesture on his part amounting to, 'You won't play; so I can't rely on you.' He felt I wasn't co-operating and was being cruel to him. However, his attitude to morphia could change dramatically. In another mood he would feel disgusted with the drug and would himself destroy it by flushing it down his lavatory. Before too long he would then feel obliged to get more drugs and indulge in a drug orgy. This contradictory behaviour signified that he was consciously not satisfied with himself or his addiction and was yet unable to tolerate the effects of being without the drug for very long. Rado (1933) noted that one way such addicts can deal with a catathymic crisis is to go into a drug-free period. In my patient, remission was too short to be effective as it was not undertaken with sufficient psychoanalytic work to enable him to work through the pain of his addictive personality towards the depressive position. Not enough of the basic restoration of the earlier, 'avoided' negotiation of life's anxieties had taken place in this particular patient. In the analytic relationship with me, I was able to recognise, only after a long time, that his vulnerability led him to treat me and the therapy as a drug which provided some relief, but a relief that did not last outside the sessions. He came to understand well that this was his way of treating me, and we both realised that we faced the complicated task of restoring a nonaddictive way of working through his problems, and of not expecting rapid results. There were many relapses in this man's treatment. It was like a game of snakes and ladders.

Francis Thompson expressed this oscillation more poetically in his poem, 'The Hound of Heaven':

*Up hopes I sped and shot precipitated*
*titanic glooms of chasmed fears.*

The destruction of progress in the treatment by acting out fluctuated considerably, but my patient's intention to recover gradually became clearer as the savagery of his internal world diminished. Eventually, this patient's analysis came to an end, once I felt that he had established a do-it-yourself outfit capable of addressing his inner conflicts. He ceased to use any prescribeable drugs but, as he later told me, turned to the regular use of alcohol, which was the addiction of his youth. He then joined Alcoholics Anonymous, working for and with them. One day he wrote to me and suggested that we should meet and have a meal together. I agreed, and I was struck by his capacity to be himself. He possessed a good degree of natural friendliness and ease of communication, which reflected some depth of character. I suspect that these strengths were acquired as a result of his having won each successive battle to overcome his problems, instead of evading them. His courage had paid dividends.

## Addiction and the superego

There are many other case histories like this one that speak of a protracted struggle to acquire the capacity to face mental pain. It is sometimes said that addicts have difficulty in this regard because of a weak superego. My experience has been the opposite: drug addicts tend to suffer under a strong and highly punitive superego. What seems to happen in addiction is that the ego is squeezed between a fierce and severe superego and the weakened ego itself, which is left to mediate a powerful id, that is, excessive infantile needs and demands which have avoided developmental processes and seek instant relief and satisfaction. The evasion of early developmental challenges, which is reflected in later evasions using drugs, can only be successfully reversed with the growth or restoration of the lost capacity to tolerate psychic pain. This is always a difficult struggle; at any given moment the drug of choice can represent the childhood mother or her surrogate and so becomes the central object of need, supplanting the virtues of human relationships. The representation the drug makes is not of the mother as a whole but rather of a part of her breast. We see this repeatedly in the clinical setting and also in literature and poetry. In Keats' 'La Belle Dame Sans Merci' the protagonist lures and seduces only to let down (see Hyatt Williams 1966). In Coleridge's *The Rime of the Ancient Mariner* (see Hyatt Williams 1986) two figures – death and life-in-death – dice for the crew of the distressed ship. Death wins the crew, and the harsh superego figure, 'life-in-death', wins the Ancient Mariner, who receives a life sentence for killing the albatross. Psychoanalytically speaking the albatross stands for the white, maternal breasts of the mother – the source of good nourishment and life processes. We know that Coleridge became addicted to opiates. Its effects were at first stimulating to his poetic career, but later on it damaged all or nearly all of his relationships. In *The Rime of the Ancient Mariner* there are several passages that suggest addiction to mood-altering and fantasy experiences. These experiences were sought by

Coleridge to contain unmanageable internal states. I would suggest that various kinds of drugs do manage to provide an initial containing experience and actually improve poetic products; however, when one might expect further development and maturity of poetic talent, the drug-taking invariably leads to considerable deterioration. This counter-productive sequence can be seen not only in creative people but also in professional and ordinary working people who take drugs. Eventually, without their drug of choice, they find it difficult to do co-ordinated work. Taking the drug does not necessarily always make things better: the work that is then achieved is liable to be unsatisfactory because the subject probably takes too little to fully assuage their anxiety and too much to be able to properly think and do what was required of them. On the one hand, we might say that the container was not effective and, on the other, the container could be so calmed down that the content was not developed properly as far as any allotted tasks were concerned.

If we consider Keats once more, he must have felt deserted by the internal image of a 'good breast-mother' at the point when his brother, Tom, died in his arms of tuberculosis. Keats dated his development of the illness to that time when he nursed, that is mothered, his sick brother only to be confronted with the death of his patient. This type of crisis is reflected in what Keats called 'The fierce dispute between damnation and impassioned clay' in his sonnet 'On Reading *King Lear* Once Again'. Psychoanalytically, this could be described as a dispute between life and death instincts, and I have found it to exist in all those addicted to hard drugs whom I have treated or assessed. Sometimes, the inevitability of death becomes recognisable quite early on in the analytic treatment. In other cases death, usually by an overdose of the selected drug, follows a considerable improvement and has the appearance of a savage annihilation of progress that the addicted patient has come to experience as an attack. The apparent ease of life to which drug addiction or habituation leads inevitably weakens and then atrophies the subject's ability to tolerate psychic pain. Hence psychic peace is procured at an increasingly high emotional price: reciprocally, the peace which is sought requires more and more of the drug of choice, or in some patients a mixture of drugs, which can produce dangerous 'cocktails' hastening the drift into mindlessness. To use Rado's term (1933), this would be the patient seeking death rather than risk being confronted by the escalation of unbearable psychic pain.

**Pharmacological effect**

It is important to note that the pharmacological effect of different drugs varies. Amphetamines can produce elation and the experience of a clear mind, but with an accompanying activity that does not exhibit wisdom.

Lysergic acid seems to dissolve the contact barrier between conscious and unconscious minds so that a curiously kaleidoscopic psychic activity occurs, reflecting the chaotic state of being in the subject. Some patients affected in this way do not recover after they have stopped using lysergic acid, and are at risk of permanent damage. It is a fact that narcotics are capable of easing or even banishing anxiety; this is their appeal. But this effect lasts for a short time only. Bion's formulations about container and contained are important in this respect, as some drugs are more containing than others. Some drugs do more damage than others, but what all drugs tend to do ultimately is to undermine and reduce, and perhaps even destroy, the adapting self of the addict in its capacity to contain and process painful states of mind. This ability tends to diminish in proportion to escalating drug use. So what begins as a viable container, albeit of a manufactured kind, loses its containing capacity and in the process depletes the addict's own capacities for containment and leaves the subject in a far worse condition than before the addiction. Of course this links with and produces the catathymic crisis described by Rado. Therapy – psychodynamic psychotherapy/psychoanalysis – slowly and with many fluctuations can, and in some patients does, reverse this situation. It is a much better catalyst to personal containment. In favourable circumstances such therapy facilitates psychic containment and psychological growth, leading to an increased capacity to contain anxieties associated with dependence upon a drug, which is essentially an unsociable type of container. The cycle of needing to feel better (that is, less or no psychic pain) only so long as the effects of the drug are operative, can be broken. A similar problem is faced with the excessive habitual use of alcohol, but this tends to have a less dramatic effect upon the personality, except where binge drinking occurs and the acute phase of intoxication is dramatic.

### The transference relationship

The transference relationship towards the psychoanalyst or psychother- apist is the crux of psychic change in the drug-dependent individual. The transference usually becomes highly ambivalent and widely polarised between idealising and demonising perspectives. These extreme points of view tend to oscillate, particularly when the tension-easing qualities of the drug are wearing off. Gradually, the psychoanalyst becomes equated with the drug, hence a fairly high frequency of relapse and acting out at breaks such as weekends or holidays. These separations generate profound anxieties in the patient for which, it is felt, no adequate container is available. In chronic addiction it is likely that the addict has suffered an inability to contain his or her needs and anxieties from the beginning, perhaps even including feelings of emptiness before being fed as an infant. At the same time, it is very difficult for the individual at risk of becoming an addict to do without the gratification which he or she has grown to expect. This situation amounts to what Bion (1967) sees as a relationship between container and contained. There develops, in situations of acute separation anxiety, an intensification of the urge to consume a substance that will assuage the demands of the 'container' part of the individual. Equally, there is a need to get rid of what cannot be tolerated by the containing part of the self in the individual who has become immersed in, and habituated to, a cycle of gratified pleasure and painful psychic content. In all cases, what is not tolerable is psychic pain. The more the drug taker is spared what James Hyatt Williams (personal communication) referred to as 'the emotional light and shade of all our days', the less able he or she will be to tolerate painful or unpleasant intrapsychic states. This is the reason why addictive illnesses tighten their hold on the individual. A vicious circle of failures to contain psychic pain – leading to increased drug use, which in turn needs to be increased as its chemical efficiency to contain pain reduces – produces an ever-worsening spiral into chronic and dangerous addiction. Rado (1933) specified the possible consequences of a 'pharmacotoxic crisis':

- flight into a drug-free period, which is a defence of a manic kind likely to collapse in subsequent states of anxiety
- suicide
- psychotic breakdown.

A feature of all three of these circumstances is a disturbed, malfunctioning relationship between container and contained. Addiction originates as an abuse of the containing part of the drug taker's psychic apparatus. As has been emphasised, the worsening of a drug-dependent condition is the consequence of a marked impairment of the psychological ability of the subject to tolerate psychic pain. It is this supplementary containing function, embodied in the drug, that the mind of the addict seeks in order to contain unbearable internal experiences. The tragedy for drug takers is that their pharmacotoxic crisis forces upon them a choice between Scylla and Charybdis similar to that which confronted the Greek sailors.

They are drawn further and further into the addiction as the drug erodes their tolerance to anxiety, alongside the immediate loss of the ability to get relief from the drug of addiction, which becomes progressively less efficient.

## Suicide

The greatest hazard to the drug addict is the risk of suicide if we follow Rado's triad of possibilities. Suicide is most likely when a catastrophic pharmacogenic crisis has occurred following the flight into a drug-free period of remission. The suicidal attempt, often ending in death itself, may be undertaken in a number of different ways. There can be a paranoid attempt, containing the implicit message: 'Look what you have done to me! This will punish you!' There may be a depressive suicide: 'Life is not worth living without drugs, and I can no longer get the relief from drugs that I used to get. I have nowhere else to turn.' An alternative depressive motivation is on the lines of: 'I want to cease upon the midnight with no pain.' A clinical variation on such suicidal impulses occurred in one addict whom I treated and who told me that, if he had a fairly long remission, the dose that he had previously been on for a while would probably kill him when he started again. Perversely, he would regard it as an athletic success if he could feel well on a dose that might kill eight men.

# Summary

The essential point of this brief chapter is to emphasise how drug-taking represents a search for a reliable container to contain the individual. The drug taker is usually a young person who is no longer able to contain himself or herself. Drug-taking does, of course, have other aetiological components; however, the desperate search for an adequate container is a primary psychological motivation. The fact that many drug-dependent individuals report and complain that central family figures were unable to provide for them the psychic containment they needed, or at least felt they needed, suggests that this is a central factor in the resort to drugs: to ease psychic pain and tension. The ongoing containment of persistent anxiety is not, however, maintained by drugs, as their effects progressively fail in this regard. More and more of the drug is taken to try to achieve containment, and this has the paradoxical and damaging effect of diminishing even further the individual's own ability to provide psychic containment and to work through psychically painful situations. These situations – intrapsychic, interpersonal or located in the external environment – become increasingly difficult to manage and the relief sought to cope with life becomes increasingly difficult to find.

Reversing this downward shift into progressive loss of containment is a major challenge to all those engaged in working with drug takers, particularly therapists who offer an alternative, more durable form of containment. The serious drug taker requires a wide range of therapeutic interventions, but, without an understanding of his or her need for containment of his or her intrapsychic condition, it will prove very difficult to reduce his or her consumption of drugs.

# CHAPTER 2

# The application of Bowlby's attachment theory to the psychotherapy of the addictions

BILL READING

## Introduction

Within the various schools of psychoanalytic thought, attachment theory is probably unsurpassed in its ability to have exerted influence upon many and diverse areas of human activity, in addition to the more routinely psychotherapeutic. It has sometimes been suggested that it was this very tendency to an interdisciplinary approach to both theory and application which helps to explain why Bowlby and his ideas were not always well-received within certain sections of the psychoanalytic community. More recently, attachment theory has assumed a secure position within the psychoanalytic world and other domains, perhaps assisted by another of its facets (and potential trigger for earlier antagonism), namely its enviable ability to lend empirical validity to its assertions.

This chapter shares with others in this volume in attempting to extend the ways in which psychodynamic ideas can be used to advance our efforts to help those with problems of addiction. Despite the widespread applications of attachment theory and its prominent position in the metapsychological world of many contemporary psychotherapists, relatively little previous attention seems to have been paid to its possible contribution to our understanding of problems of addiction and their psychotherapeutic management.

Bowlby and his followers have posited that the attachment dynamic is a universal characteristic of the interpersonal relationships of humans and some other animal species. The attachment needs and dynamics of both patient and therapist are inevitably implicated in the psychotherapeutic encounter. The nature and extent of the involvement of the attachment dynamics of patient and therapist will clearly vary from one therapy to another and even from one session to another within a particular therapy.

Also, therapists are likely to vary considerably in their tendency to make both private and overt reference to such dynamics. Psychotherapy may be conducted with no conscious reference to attachment theory, though it can be argued that the attachment dynamic will be inevitably and often crucially implicated in the process of therapy.

Another theme of this volume is to invite the reader to consider those modifications of approach and technique that will assist in providing helpful psychotherapy to our addicted patients. Attachment theory can be seen as influencing the practice of therapy in two main ways (Mackie 1981). First, the therapeutic alliance is regarded as a situation in which the therapist functions as a temporary attachment figure, providing the client with a secure base from which he or she becomes enabled to embark on the exploratory work of therapy – a situation that has been described as being analogous to the one in which the securely attached infant is able to play and explore the environment when in proximity to the mother, or other figure with whom a satisfactory attachment bond has been established. Second, the transference relationship becomes one in which maladaptive aspects of the patient's relationship (that is insecure patterns of attachment) with the therapist can be identified and worked through. Such insecure patterns are regarded as strategies that have been associated with viability when deployed in the conduct of past relationships and which are thus being repeated in present relationships with others, including that with the therapist. Of course, the secure-base and transference-analysis components must be viewed in the context of their recursive interaction. More particularly, transference-analysis becomes indicated at those points where (usually negative) transference distortions temporarily compromise the secure-base experience and, thus, the capacity for further exploratory work.

The ability to engage in the kind of 'confidence-relationship' (Benedek 1938) that is paradigmatic of 'attachment proper' represents a goal towards which we may be seen as encouraging our patients to move. Viewed this way, much of the work of therapy comprises the working through of those defences, resistances and other obstacles that combine to maintain the restrictive yet predictable modes of relationship predicated on certain 'insecure' configurations of the Internal Working Models (IWM, see p. 17). It will be argued also that the work of therapy may be extended to include the working through of the (homeostatic) relationship which has been established between the patient and the drug(s) of choice.

Attachment-based therapy shares with other modalities within psychotherapy in its attempts to enhance the patient's ability to locate his or her symptoms in an interpersonal context. Particular emphasis is placed on the ability to achieve improved 'narrative competence' – a more coherent, concise and helpful account of one's personal history. It is the quality of narrative competence that serves as one of the most important indicators of the success or otherwise of such therapy and which is found to be positively correlated with secure attachment (Main et al 1985) and in turn, personal attributes such as ego-resilience, autonomous functioning and the capacity to establish secure relationships with others (Sroufe 1979).

Attachment-based psychotherapy to likely to be conducted within an alliance that provides a supportive milieu in which exploratory work can take place and may, thus, be seen as suited to the needs of a client group which is unlikely to benefit from overly expressive techniques, particularly in the earlier stages of therapy (Ball and Legow 1996).

Additionally, this chapter offers two assertions. First, that the patient's relationship with the drug(s) may be seen as being imbued with some of those characteristics which have been so well demonstrated in interpersonal relationships from the purview of attachment theory. Secondly, that the inclusion of this perspective has clinical usefulness. Perhaps one of the most important sources of its usefulness derives from a potential expansion of the therapist's empathic repertoire and the associated capacity to achieve high levels of acclimatisation and responsiveness to the patient's experiences and particularly to the relationship with the drug(s) of choice.

The tendency of psychodynamicists and others to use dependency-based models of addiction may lead us to overlook the crucial differences that may exist in the appreciation between the instrumental/secondary nature of the (dependent) need to procure supply (for example food, tension-discharge or self-esteem) and the primary quality of the need for attachment which exists not as a means to an end but as an end in itself.

In practice, of course, the infant's sense of security (derived from proximity to the attachment figure) is likely to exist in conflation with experiences of need-satisfaction, which derive from the relationship with the same object – the infant will experience mother as both providing safety and as a source of pleasurable gratification. Similarly, it is proposed here that the relationship between the drug user and the drug itself may be associated with experiences both of security and of the satisfaction of needs as a result of its chemical and symbolic effects.

*I started to feel better the moment I knew I was going to buy some booze. On the way to the off licence, my hands were shaking. I wasn't withdrawing; it was sheer excitement ... and anticipation ... yeah, anticipation. (Anon)*

It is the aim here to give sufficient details of attachment theory to enable a consideration of its role in the addictive processes. It will not be possible here to give a detailed summary of attachment theory or of the ways in which the theory may become a useful additional metaphor in the study of addiction-specific psychotherapy. Where necessary, the reader is urged to undertake additional reading which will permit a better understanding of the theory, critiques of the theory and its application to psychotherapy – both general and addiction-specific (for example Holmes 1993). What follows is a brief summary of some of the central features of attachment theory as a prelude to a consideration of its relevance within the addictions.

## The central tenets of attachment theory

### 1. The need for proximity and the secure-base

Bowlby suggests that humans and members of some other animal species manifest an innate tendency to seek and maintain proximity to certain preferred others. Unlike the phenomenon of imprinting in some species, patterns of attachment are observed to be cultivated over time, giving rise to differing relationships with specific and distinct others. Bowlby employs the term 'affectional-bond' (Bowlby 1979) to describe the developing attachment – a term that allows a clear contrast to be made between the ambience of the attachment relationship and that of the instrumentalism of need-driven dependencies.

Where the infant is able to enjoy proximity to an attachment figure who is attuned to its inner world and responsive to its emotional and other modes of expression, secure-base experience becomes possible. When experiencing secure-base provision, the infant will not be anxious, will engage in exploratory play and will be relatively unconcerned with any need to focus attention upon the proximity or responsiveness of the attachment figure. It is as if sufficient repetition of experiences of secure-base provision will incline the developing child to be able to take for granted that the caregiver is present and that her or his responsiveness can be safely assumed, should the need arise. The consistent experience of such reliable relationship episodes provides the basis for internalisations, which, in turn, form the basis for a propensity to seek out others with whom similar confidence-relationships may be replicated (see Internal Working Models on p. 17).

### 2. Homeostasis

Attachment theory suggests that the attached couple(s) will collaborate in strategies which combine to maintain the status quo of the relationship and to preserve it from external threat to its persistence. Such strategies range from the <u>behavioural</u> (for example living in close geographical proximity), <u>perceptual</u> (for example the 'defensive exclusion' of experiences that might be contradictory to the state of the relationship) to the <u>interpersonal</u> protocols by which the couple become adept at relating in such a way as to promote attainment of the 'set goal' of proximity.

I suggest later that it is helpful to extend our models of the resistances to include a form of attachment-resistance – a situation in which our therapeutic interventions are met with opposition arising from the threat that our attempts to be helpful may pose to the patient's object relationships, including those between client and drug(s).

### 3. The quality of experience and the Internal Working Models (IWM)

Attachment theory offers a particular view of object-relatedness in which actual experiences with others become internally represented and form a template for the conduct of some future relationships. The qualities and attributes of relationships with significant others will be replicated in the 'internalised memories of experiences in relationship' (IMERs) (Heard and Lake 1986), with the IMERs, in turn, disposing the individual to seek opportunities to engage in relationships in which their prototypic configurations will be repeated. The IMERs may be relatively secure or insecure – in either case, they are likely to reflect the quality of previously experienced relationship episodes.

Attachment researchers have been able to demonstrate a strong tendency for the observed quality of relationships between one-year-old infants and their caregivers to be directly predictive of their later personal attributes, including attachment-pattern categorisation, style of interpersonal relating and ego-competencies.

### 4. Hierarchy of Internal Working Models

An individual is seen as having internal representations of relationships with past or current important others, with these representations being organised hierarchically. For the infant, it is the mother or other principal caregiver whose representation is likely to occupy a position at the head of the hierarchy, just as it is she whose proximity the infant will seek at times of danger or stress. It is posited that the internal hierarchical organisation of the IMERs can be seen as undergoing revision across the life cycle, though the rate and extent of such revision will generally decline in tandem with ageing and maturity. While it has sometimes been argued that attachment theory may lose some of its relevance when applied to adult–adult relationships, others have suggested that the processes involved continue though with qualitative and quantitative distinctions from those at work in relationships with infants. For example, Weiss (1982) suggests that adult–adult attachments will manifest less discrepancy between levels of mastery, be more equal and that they will be more likely to include mutual sexual components than infant–adult bonds.

## 5. The attachment behavioural system

Attachment-behaviour is the term used to describe those interpersonal, subjective and behavioural strategies that are employed by the attached couple in order to preserve/re-establish secure-base conditions when these are subject to perceived danger or when separation is threatened/ occurs. Such strategies include distress vocalisations, increased autonomic arousal/anxiety, clinging and searching. It is important to understand that attachment-behaviour is not active when secure-base conditions obtain. It is when attachment bonds are under stress that the attachment behavioural system is activated and when other behavioural systems correspondingly deactivate. Reunion after separation and/or the passing of any perceived danger is associated with the deactivation of the attachment behavioural system and a concomitant reactivation of those other systems that have become suspended in the service of the re-establishment of the secure-base. For example, the securely attached infant is likely to manifest little overt attention to the attachment-figure when in her/his proximity and may engage in exploratory play. The experience of potential threat or separation will be likely to activate the attachment behavioural system, for example in the form of crying, clinging and searching, and play will become suspended (deactivated). Cessation of a perceived threat/separation will result in a brief engagement in reassuring/comforting behaviours as the attachment behavioural system deactivates and other systems (that is, play) reactivate. Homeostasis has been restored and another successful relationship episode becomes available for potential internalisation (see Figure 2.1).

## 6. Moving on, loss and the working through of endings

As an experimental/experiential test of the theory, it can be a helpful exercise to compose lists of the relationships that have been of most importance at various stages in one's life thus far (for example infancy, childhood, adolescence, early adulthood, etc.) and to consider the themes and patterns which emerge as a result. It is likely that the experiment will reveal that changes in relationship configurations will be seen as having usually occurred gradually with the individual engaging in progressively longer absences from former attachment-figures as she/he makes an increasing commitment to new others of significance. Changes in the internal hierarchy of IMERs may be seen as occurring incrementally, via a gradual process of adjustment. For the securely attached individual, prolonged separation (particularly as a consequence of sudden/perceived loss) from the attachment figure will initiate *separation distress*. The bereft partner mourns the loss of the loved other and in so doing is able to accomplish two major goals. First, successful mourning will allow the IWM of the relationship to become a viable inner source of persisting assuagement and, second, the individual becomes able to form new attachments. Clearly, the notion of a grieving process and of its proper resolution becomes a vital requirement for successful survival of loss and especially for the ability to forge new affectional bonds.

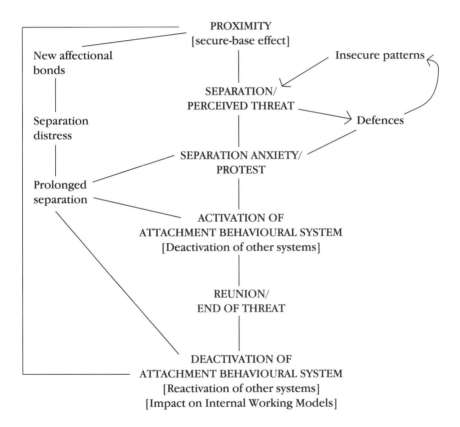

**Figure 2.1:** A model of the attachment behavioural system. The pathway to the left of the central column depicts the satisfactory movement back to a position of proximity/secure-base. To the right is depicted the possible route of entry into defensive/insecure patterns of attachment. Note that progress on both left and right routes forms the basis for a further impact on the organisation of Internal Working Models. Note also the recursive interplay between attachment and other behavioural systems.

## Addiction and attachment

Central to the definition of addictions is the observation that the individual repeats some piece of (harmful) behaviour in apparent contradiction to subjective and/or objective desires that such repetition should not occur. The addicted individual will often report and/or be perceived as being subject to compulsive elements that lead him or her to repeat apparently unwanted behaviour. Many hypotheses have been offered in an attempt to explain the nature of this type of behaviour, ranging from those that view the addict as a hapless victim of disease or other processes beyond conscious control through to those models that regard addiction as comprising nothing more than a socially constructed explanation which allows the addict and/or others to obscure and mystify the conscious decision to use drugs in ways which are considered to be harmful etc. What is to follow comprises an invitation to the reader to consider the role of the attachment dynamic in contributing to the incidence and persistence of such phenomena.

Rather than offering an explanatory hypothesis, the aim is to create an additional vantage point from which the intricacies of some patients' relationships with their drug(s) may be viewed, particularly via their transferential manifestations and also within the more general psychotherapeutic setting.

## Attachment and Zinberg's Tripartite Model

The adoption of a perspective derived from attachment theory gives rise to specific observations and possibilities for the understanding of the psychotherapeutic process in application to the addictions. Perhaps most prominent amongst these is the view that our patients may establish affectional bonds with their drugs of choice and that the relationship with the therapist needs to be regarded as being initiated within the context of the pre-existing relationship between patient and drug. More subtly, attachment theory offers a particular means of understanding the way in which the therapist engages in the process of therapy and of how a triangulation between therapist, patient and drug may be observed – especially in regard to the transference relationship.

Zinberg's Tripartite Model of Compulsive Drug Use (Zinberg 1975) offers a convenient way in which some of the interplay between addictive behaviour and attachment can be considered. This model proposes that compulsive drug use may be understood as being usefully conceptualised as arising from the interaction between three components, namely the *drug*, the *set* and the *setting*.

## 1. *The drug*

The drug may be seen as being valued for its intrinsic (that is, pharmaco-logical) effects and for its (inevitably related) symbolic meaning to the individual. Just as the emotional life and anxiety level of the infant become highly contingent upon the relationship with the attachment figure, so the drug user may be seen as becoming progressively more likely to regulate feeling and anxiety through the use of the drug. In some instances, it is clearly the directly experienced effect of the drug (for example anxiety reduction, stimulation) that is most important to a particular user. Many patients will present with histories of difficulty in establishing collaborative relationships with others and the use of drugs is commonly interwoven into such relationships that exist. If one considers the high-risk situations that are found repeatedly to be associated with lapses and relapses, it seems that negative emotional states consistently figure amongst those factors which precede the decision to revert to increased levels of drug use. This may be seen as analogous to the situation in which the infant turns to the attachment figure at times of particular stress in order to re-establish proximity and to receive reassuring and comforting responses in the process. The drug may be seen as offering a chemical means of achieving similar subjective consequences to those derived from the infant's reunion with mother at times of difficulty. For example, it has been suggested that drugs may be used in order to provide functions which are deficient within the ego, with this very deficiency resulting, in turn, from the failure to have inter-nalised sufficient experiences of having been cared for by others in infancy (for example, Kohut 1977a) The (literal) incorporation of the drug constitutes a means by which missing psychic function may be (omnipotently) replaced. For others, it seems that the drug serves as a surrogate for needed yet unavailable/shunned others and that this form of surrogacy may be(come) preferred to the relative precariousness of attempts to relate to human others. In considering the application of attachment theory to such perspectives, further emphasis is given to the way in which the relationship between the drug and its taker may be understood, particularly the way in which this relationship becomes represented in the second of Zinberg's dimensions – namely the *set*.

## 2. *The set*

'There is no such thing as an addict. Wherever one looks, one sees the couple formed of the addict and his or her drug(s) of choice.' This corruption of Winnicott's (1964) famous assertion is offered as a means of acknowledging the tendency of the addicted patient to have become increasingly identified with his or her drug(s) both in the eyes of others and, more crucially, within the world of internal object relations, composed of representations of the self (user), the other (drug) and the interaction of self and other, respectively (the user in relation to the drug). A form of Internal Working Model is laid down through repeated experiences of the recourse to the drug(s) and it is to such internalisations that the addict will subtly refer during routine (that is, not excessively stressful) episodes in order to derive a sense of security. When stressors are such as to exceed the usual parameters associated with homeostasis, recourse to the drug(s) will be correspondingly more pronounced. Such recourse is likely to occur both in the form of its internal representation (for example craving, increased thoughts/fantasies about the drug or its use) and may also be subject to literal enactments in the form of resumption of use, heavier use, etc.

In keeping with the findings of attachment theory, it should be noted that attachment behaviour per se becomes increasingly activated at times characterised by the experience of danger and/or threat to the affectional bond itself. Conversely, attachment behaviour becomes deactivated at times when such perceived threat is absent. Thus it may be the case that aspects of the addicted client's set in regard to the drug become active (and thus available for exploration/working through) under similar conditions – that is, danger and/or threat to the relationship with the drug. Few who offer therapy to addicted clients will be unfamiliar with the situation in which apparently motivated, sincere and insightful clients nevertheless lapse/relapse. In subsequent sessions, the clients themselves are often at a loss to account for the apparent discrepancy between their statements of intent and their actions.

Further, such clients often express the view that previous awareness of high-risk situations, probable adverse consequences, etc. had not disappeared but had seemed to become less immediate, seemingly eclipsed by a predominating focus on the drug(s). Coinciding with the heightened emphasis on the drug is a deactivation of other perceptual and behavioural systems, perhaps most especially those that might potentially counter the activation of systems geared towards re-establishing proximity to the drug(s). Cognitive-behavioural (CB) approaches have encouraged the use of interventions that help clients to identify and modify those modes of thought which can be seen as likely to lead to increased incidences of lapse and relapse. In doing so, we try to assist the client in maintaining a cognitive vigilance towards internal and external cues and other antecedents to drug use. However, it is probable that two of the assumptions of the CB approach will differ significantly from that that which derives from attachment theory.

First, lapsing is likely to be conceptualised as being more likely to occur where the client undergoes reduced vigilance, experiences low self-efficacy, has a poor range of available coping strategies, etc. In other words, the CB approach places emphasis on the deficiency of those attributes that can be seen as having become deactivated in the service of a reorientation to the drug. Techniques within the CB model are organised in an attempt to redress the resultant deficits through reframing, skills training, etc. Such strategies may be of great help to the client as a means of reducing the risk of relapse, but it is clear that clients frequently report that periods of craving seem often to be characterised by an escalating focus of the fantasy and anticipation of resumed drug use in which alternative strategies etc. cease to be central. Thus craving is more likely to be viewed as an expression of the activation of systems that act in concert so as to facilitate reunion with the drug and which actively exclude other systems whose aim may be seen as attempting to avert the prospect of relapse/reunion. Rather than attributing lapsing to low self-efficacy, attachment theory allows for the inclusion of an increasing sense of efficacy (that is, in the form of both ability to use the drug and also the anticipation of its effects in facilitating increased competencies) which is predicated on internalisations of past, repeated episodes in which the client's use of the drug has been experienced as providing a variant of secure-base, particularly at times of increased anxiety/threat.

Second, in common with many other models, the deficit hypothesis of the CB approach tends to consign fantasised or actual drug use to the role of symptom/unwanted behaviour and risks omitting to note its more positive connotation in the client's schemata. There is a good deal of evidence that the therapist's capacity for empathy represents an important variable in engaging and retaining clients in treatment, in both substance-misuse-specific and generic therapy. The therapist's lack of empathy with the addictional bond (between client and drug[s]) may give rise to a rather lopsided posture in which the therapist aligns with the client's wish to bring about change but fails to acknowledge aspects of the conflictive nature of the patient's dilemma. The potential for the therapist's disavowal of aspects of the patient's experience may be increased by adherence to models of addiction therapy that discourage emphasis of the positive components of drug-use experiences (for example the cautionary attitude to 'stinking thinking' within some 'Twelve-step Fellowship' programmes) or by more idiosyncratic counter-transference reactions, as in the following example from a group-therapy session.

*Tom*

> *Tom has been describing the difficulty he has in staying off alcohol for more*
> *than short periods.*
> *Tom: I don't know what it is. I know that I've got to stop drinking, and I want*
> *to stop because of all the problems it always causes ... I know I can't carry on,*
> *but then I get sort of scared ... and I don't know if I can do it.*
> *Therapist: Perish the thought of life without alcohol, eh, Tom?*
> *(Tom remains silent, some other group members smile, the discussion moves*
> *on to apparently unrelated matters.)*
> *In a subsequent supervision session the therapist was able to explore his*
> *hostile reaction towards Tom, whom he had experienced as 'whinging about*
> *the loss of a drug' while he (the therapist) had been required to cope with*
> *important (and unsatisfactorily unresolved) bereavement.*

## 3. The setting

Zinberg regarded the setting as comprising the most important element in
the Tripartite Model in its contribution to the aetiology of compulsive drug
use. It has been the emphasis on the quality of interactions within the
setting that has informed the development of contemporary treatment
modes such as motivational enhancement therapy, relapse prevention
therapy and others which draw heavily upon the principles of social
learning theory.

Central to Bowlby's work on attachment theory is the view that the
need for relationships with others is driven by innate need and that it is
the vicissitudes of experiences in and of the relationship which will
determine the pathway through which such needs will be expressed in
the future. Many addicts are likely to present with histories of apparently
disordered relationships. It is often the case that the social network will
be composed of others with similar drug-taking habits and the prospect
of recovery may often confront the addicts with the realisation that social
networks are contingent upon continued drug use and also that recovery
will necessitate alterations in lifestyle, acquaintances, etc. Drug use may
serve as an indispensable symbol of membership of the particular
subgroup and the chemical and symbolic effects of the drug(s) may
provide the user with such disinhibition, stimulation, etc. as is necessary
to facilitate social interaction within, and sometimes outside of the
subgroup. A reduction/cessation of drug use may threaten the individual
with social isolation, which may persist for long periods while the process
of establishing alternative networks takes place. Perhaps one of the most
important functions for the therapeutic setting is to provide the potentially alienated addict with the opportunity for surrogate, temporary
attachments during the hiatus that may occur between the suspension of
relationships which are contingent on continued drug use and the estab-

lishment of an alternative social network. Those treatment modalities that offer the opportunity for shared experience which is not contingent upon continued drug use (for example group therapy, Concept Houses, Fellowship programmes) provide the most obvious means of providing substitute, and sometimes, lifelong sources of social interaction. Within such settings, conversation/interaction will often centre around references to drug use and closely related issues, and this focus seems often to represent a means by which the drug(s) may be kept within proximity and continue in its role as enabler of social affiliations, however paradoxically:

> We recognised that we were powerless over alcohol and that our lives had become unmanageable. (Step One, Alcoholics Anonymous)
> You just can't talk to people outside these groups in the same way ... they wouldn't be able to understand. (Participant in group-therapy programme for addicted clients)

The individual therapist may also be able to provide the client with an alternative relationship to that with the drug(s) of choice. Indeed, in some instances it seems possible to detect the way in which the client's gradually developing attachment to the therapist is paralleled by his or her increasing ability to tolerate progressively longer absences from the drug(s) – perhaps in keeping with Bowlby's contention that the therapist should function as a temporary attachment figure for the patient in therapy. As the restrictive and destructive bond(age) to the drug becomes reduced, the patient becomes progressively more enabled to use the security of the therapeutic situation as a base from which more ambitious exploration of his or her position becomes possible and with it the prospect of more adaptive coping mechanisms.

> She took no medication at all on those mornings [of therapy] and would arrive feeling pretty ill, but always by the end of the session felt much better and found that a 'person' was better than a 'pill', a highly important discovery for her, for she had been under heavy medication for years. (Guntrip 1969, p. 338)

Guntrip's description of the patient's discovery reveals his commitment to a crucial premise in some schools of psychotherapy – specifically, the conviction that it is the move towards the interpersonal/intersubjective experiencing, exploration and resolution of personal difficulty which informs the course of the therapeutic process and dialogue. The therapist's capacity to commit to such a view of therapy will be mediated by factors including those which I will review in the concluding section of this chapter, in which I consider some of the implications for the therapist in attempting to employ attachment theory when conducting psychotherapy, especially with addicted clients.

## Some considerations for the addictions therapist employing attachment theory

### 1. The alliance is therapeutic

Attachment-based psychotherapy belongs to the supportive school of psychotherapeutic thought. The therapist aims to establish a good working alliance with the client, a situation analogous to a mother's ability to offer her infant secure-base provision. In both situations, the patient/infant is able to engage in greater exploration and play. Rather paradoxically, it is the ability to experience intimacy in a safe environment that provides the basis for the achievement of a viable sense of autonomy, with the resultant autonomy paving the way for an enhanced capacity to enjoy intimacy and so on.

Since it is assumed that the range and quality of the patient's Internal Working Models remain open to adaptation, therapy proceeds on the basis that the positively experienced alliance will, itself, become internalised and with it the capacity for the patient to draw on reorganised and improved templates for the conduct of future relationships and the revision of those already in existence – including the relationship with the drug(s) of choice.

The attachment-based therapist is likely to be less concerned to interpret the transference than his or her more conventionally psychoanalytic colleague, with the important exception of doing so at those points where defensive patterns of anxious attachment threaten to disrupt the secure-base experience. In keeping with the emphasis on the *positive alliance*, interpretation is offered in a supportive (rather than a regressive) atmosphere. The patient's tendency to resort to defensiveness when relating to the therapist is responded to in the context of the understanding and resolution of whatever it is that may have disturbed his or her sense of security within the alliance. For a useful discussion of some of the ways in which the therapist may adapt posture and technique within the supportive modes of therapy see Holmes (1996). It is perhaps worth pausing to reflect on the fact that the therapist's own Internal Working Models are also subject to revision as a result of experiences within a relationship, including those with patients. It is to be hoped that the therapist's own internal and external worlds are such as to enable him or her to function as a consistent-enough attachment figure so that the work of therapy is able to proceed relatively free of the therapist's need to use the therapeutic encounter to work through/enact his or her own attachment anxieties. As with other therapeutic modes that place greater emphasis on the therapist being present, case-supervision, a period of personal therapy, the stability of the therapist's personal relationships and the support of colleagues are among those factors which help to ensure that it is the best interests of the patient (as opposed to the unresolved needs of the therapist) which inform the framing and delivery of the therapist's interventions. Of course, supervision, itself, can be readily modelled upon the secure-base model.

## 2. Therapy threatens the addictional bond

Many addicted clients realise or come to recognise that reduction/ cessation of drug use is essential if meaningful personal change is to be possible; few, if any, have not acknowledged this prior to seeking help to change. It was the observation that the bond with the drug often resisted attempts to change it which first triggered my own interest in the way in which this bond seemed to conform to at least some of the underlying principles that had derived from the study of person-to-person affectional bonds.

Psychotherapists and others engaged in offering help to addicted clients are clearly in a position in which they are implicitly and often explicitly identified with the prospect of drug reduction/cessation. Attachment theory may offer a helpful metaphor for understanding and, importantly, empathising with some of the transferential manifestations of the client's resultant transferential ambivalence. Missed appointments, deceit and various other modes of defensiveness can be usefully appre-hended as deriving from the patient's attempt to negotiate the relationship with a figure who simultaneously represents both a trusted ally in the pursuit of change and a despised, potential threat to the homeostasis of the bond with the drug of choice.

## 3. The ambivalent transference needs working through

The patient's ambivalent experience of the therapist as helper/depriver may manifest itself in numerous ways. The expression of the patient's opposition to the therapist's ministrations will often be expressed indirectly, though frequently with the potential to create powerful countertransference feelings, such as hopelessness, impotence, anger or the tendency to persecutory-retaliatory interpretation.

The therapist who is role-secure is more likely to be able to respond to potential provocation of this kind in terms of offering empathic under-standing of its meaning within the patient's struggle to reconcile the conflicting demands for change on one hand and homeostasis on the other. Wurmser (1978) suggests that it is the patient's tendency to enact his or her internal drama, via the process of 'externalisation', which provides the therapist with a source of highly fertile clinical material. The therapist's capacity both to take the transference and to use the counter-transference under such conditions enables the patient's projected ambivalence to the relationship with the drug itself to be explored in vivo as interpretative links are made between the dramas enacted with the therapist and the patient's inner world. The role-secure therapist is able to manifest a vital combination of attached concern and non-attached curiosity as he or she witnesses the enactment of the patient's dilemmas. This requires a skilful admixture of qualities on the part of the therapist.

### 4. Attachment behaviour is activated under conditions of threat

Given that the attachment behavioural system is activated at times of excessive stress and/or when affectional bonds are under threat, it would seem to follow that behavioural systems geared to the maintenance of proximity to the drug will also become activated when the addictional bond is threatened. The emergence of apparently countertherapeutic phenomena during the course of therapy, such as craving, hoarding/clinging, seemingly irrelevant decisions, etc. may alarm both therapist and patient alike. Rather than necessarily providing evidence of either the patient's lack of motivation or the therapist's incompetence, such occurrences may be seen as encouraging (though somewhat paradoxical) signs that dynamic change may be in process. The absence of manifest *attachment resistance* may be seen as evidence that the addic-tional bond is free from threat! Once again, the therapist's capacity to offer empathic understanding of the basis for such attachment resistance may be crucial in influencing whether or not its creative therapeutic potential is realised.

As a footnote to the question of interpretation of transferential ambiva-lence, I find it helpful to remind myself of the communicative function of emotion and anxiety within attachment theory and related interpersonal psychologies. Within such disciplines, the expression of emotion and anxiety is more likely to be viewed as constituting a means by which the individual attempts to evoke a response from the other. For the therapist working with addicted clients, the patient's expressions of this kind may provide clues to the need for an attuned response. For example, the emergence of hostile feelings towards the therapist may reflect the patient's insecurity as the bond with the drug becomes subject to explo-ration during therapy. Under such circumstances, the therapist who, for example, needs to be liked by patients may experience difficulty in holding (in mind) the patient's deeper experience.

## 5. The therapist models the capacity to let go

As stated earlier, drug use may have provided the user with both the direct and indirect means by which needs for companionship have been assuaged and/or facilitated, albeit defensively (Heard and Lake 1986). Cessation/reduction of drug use invites the potential to experience loss of both proximity to the drug itself and of those relationships/social networks to which drug use has facilitated membership in the past. Since the process of mourning losses seems to be crucial in freeing the bereaved individual to form new attachments (and to relinquish ties to old ones) the therapist needs to be able to acknowledge and facilitate the patient's need to grieve such losses where appropriate.

Therapists may be prone to forms of resistance in which defensive exclusion is employed to avoid the acknowledgement of material that poses a potential threat to the homeostasis which has been established with a particular patient. The potential for such a threat may be posed by the possibilities of both relapse and of symptom reduction, the patient's changing requirements of the alliance and, ultimately, the patient's need to terminate therapy. The ability of the therapist to let go as appropriate can be seen as central within many schools of psychotherapy but assumes particular importance within the attachment paradigm as the therapist works to maintain an attitude of non-attachment both to the patients' productions and to the patients themselves. Therapy may provide the patient with an unprecedented opportunity to discover that the relationship is possible in the absence of attitudes of possessiveness and clinging, for example, and not only that the experience of separation can be managed but also that it may pave the way for new possibilities.

## 6. The role of the supervisor

It has often been my experience that the therapist's response to supervision can provide a useful source of data in which the parallel process operates so as to mirror aspects of the therapist/patient and patient/drug triads. Failed tape-recordings of sessions, lost notes and other modes of 'amnesia' may sometimes be usefully explored in their role as forms of defensive exclusion to experiences that hold the potential to threaten the respective homeostases of patient/drug, therapist/patient and supervisor/ supervisee.

I consider that the attachment-based supervisor aims to provide a supportive space in which the supervisee is able to enjoy an ambience similar to that discussed above when considering the requirements of secure-base provision. In common with good supervision deriving from other theoretical schools, I assume that both supervisor and supervisee

take responsibility for behaving ethically and honestly. These are fundamental requirements for a creative relationship of this kind, and
attachment theory offers a shared metaphor under the aegis of which such
a relationship may prosper.

# CHAPTER 3

# The vulnerable self: Heinz Kohut and the addictions

MARTIN WEEGMANN

The work of Heinz Kohut has had a major impact on the development of psychoanalytic ideas, notably in America, and has led to the school of Self Psychology. There are important crossover points between his ideas and those of a number of British analysts, particularly those associated with the Independent tradition, with Balint and Winnicott as good examples. Differences in language and tradition may, of course, obscure some of these similarities in both clinical emphasis and theory.

At its most general, Kohut has offered us a new theory of the self and its development, highlighting many aspects of both normal and pathological narcissism. As is well known, Kohut argued that pejorative and morally tinged attitudes have influenced and handicapped a true understanding of narcissism in psychoanalysis, which has frequently been seen as part of some early stage to be replaced or grown out of by object relations. At an analytic and an everyday level it carries regrettable overtones of selfishness or self-centredness. In his view, by contrast, there are separate and equally legitimate lines of development of both narcissistic aspects of the character as well as object love. Narcissism is not outgrown, though in its development there is a gradual transformation from more global and primitive narcissism to more mature forms of self-investment and self-sustenance. The ability to achieve the latter, a state that Fairbairn (1943/1952) might have, in different language, described as one of 'mature dependence' or Bowlby (1988a) as one of healthy 'self-reliance', is a major constituent of the sense of security in oneself and the ability to cope in adult life.

Kohut developed his ideas through the treatment of patients with narcissistic personality disorder, where he felt that a traditional psychoanalytic approach had made little headway. Although he did not work with addictions, he nevertheless thought that there was some affinity between such a personality disorder and the *acting out* disorders: addiction, delinquency and perversion. Given his shift from placing centrality on the instincts, he reclassified these areas not as merely impulse disorders but rather as primary disorders of the self. In a primary disorder of the self, there is an assumption that the individual has a major, and not temporary, difficulty in building a sense of self-cohesion or maintaining sufficient self-esteem or vigour.

Curiously, just as Kohut moved away from classical Freudian ideas to his own self psychology, so in the history of psychodynamic thinking about the addictions there has been a comparable transition from the early analysts, with their emphasis on libido theory, oral dependence and regressive attachment to drugs, to later views, emphasising the importance of ego deficits and the regulation of affect. It is suggested here that this shift in perspective can open up a less critical, more accepting view of the narcissistic vulnerability in addicted individuals and of the adaptive functions which the drug serves for the ego. Clearly, these adaptive or protective aspects of drug-taking are difficult for the outsider faced with the devastating negative consequences of the addiction to comprehend and perhaps can only be appreciated by a careful, though not collusive, exploration of how the drugs fit into the client's internal world. Considerable skills of empathy are needed.

Rather than systematically applying Kohut's complicated ideas to addiction, I have instead chosen to identify a number of areas where, in my view, his work offers a helpful or novel perspective. Following an excursion into theory, I have drawn on two clinical examples from individual psychotherapy, my supervisory work with other professionals and examples of the kind of countertransference pressures that arise. This is limited and makes no attempt, for example, to consider how his views might have differing relevance according to different stages of recovery, from detoxification through to more advanced sobriety, or, indeed, maintenance treatments for drug users; the interested reader is referred to the excellent 'three-phase psychotherapeutic method' of Kaufman (1994), drawing on self-psychology and several other models, and Levin's (1987) book, offering a specific application of Kohut's ideas to the process of recovery. Owing to the constraints of space, it is not possible to comment on how Fellowship organisations – like AA, NA and others – help to modify the problematic narcissism of people in recovery and, in particular, harness the power of group affiliation to address vulnerabilities in self-governance and self-regulation (see Khantzian and Mack's 1989 outstanding contribution).

## Theory

In Kohut's theory, patients who are narcissistically orientated and vulnerable have chronic problems in maintaining a normal level of self-esteem and are highly sensitive to slights, rejections or perceived criticism. This may be apparent in vulnerable-looking, thin-skinned patients who are easily bruised, but it also applies less directly in those narcissistic individuals whose character armouring involves arrogance, vanity or other postures of invulnerability. Fried (1979) suggests that the main difference between these broad groups is that the former patients display their wounds more visibly and may present as victims, while the latter display strong narcissistic defences and project outwardly in an effort to rid the self of any feelings of vulnerability. Traditional psychoanalysis, with its emphasis on drives, defences and libidinal conflicts proved problematic with narcissistic patients, leading Kohut and others to investigate the emergence of specific narcissistic needs through treatment, which had to be approached quite differently from those involving other kinds of mental conflict. He spoke of the emergence of particular kinds of 'narcissistic transference', or, using his later terminology, 'selfobject transferences' in which the analyst is experienced as providing a basic function or an extension of the self.

To start with, he enumerated two main kinds of such transference: (a) the 'mirror transference' (with various subdivisions), which is activated through experiences of insufficiently supported childhood needs for acceptance and responsive mirroring by the parents and (b) the 'idealising transference', which is activated from the child's need to feel part of a source of idealised strength and calmness, which an admired parent provides. Kohut progressively formulated the concept of 'selfobjects', by which he meant an experience of objects that are felt to be part of the self and over whom we expect control. Two kinds of 'selfobject' correspond to these two transference patterns, which are (1) those selfobjects that notice and confirm the child's vigour or greatness, known as 'mirroring selfob-jects' and (2) selfobjects that the child can in turn admire and feel part of, sharing in the calm or infallibility which they represent, known as the 'idealised parent imago'.

The self is a complex achievement rather than an endowment, built up successively though innumerable interactions with our carers in the past, who are significant to us because they not only meet our physical needs but also function as our selfobjects, responding continually to our psychological needs. Drawing an analogy to the body's need for oxygen, Kohut regards the need for responsive selfobjects to be no less essential for normal mental growth and balance – in his words, 'the child is born (or should be) into an empathic responsive human milieu (of selfobjects) ... he "expects" it' (1977a, p. 85). A serious deficiency in the availability or quality of such selfobjects will produce, in mental terms, the equivalent to the body being gradually starved of physical nutrients. A cohesive and confident self emerges, by contrast, from an optimal relationship between a child and his or her selfobjects, allowing for normal imperfections and frustrations of parenting to be fully integrated. This is akin to Winnicott's (1947) 'ordinary devoted' or 'good enough' mother, and throughout normal development there will be 'the gradual replacement of the selfobjects and their functions by a self and *its* functions' (my emphasis, Kohut and Wolf 1978, p. 418). In other words, the self is able to perform the regulating, soothing, accepting and motivating functions that it was previously dependent on others to provide.

In adult life a sufficiently cohesive and secure self helps the individual to tolerate normal fluctuations in self-esteem and so to cope with ordinary rejections, disappointments, obstacles and achievements. In other words, we develop a normal, though not omnipotent, capacity to withstand the slings and arrows of outrageous fortune without buckling to it. Kohut believes that we never outgrow our need for mirroring and idealisable selfobjects; these have a different quality in adult life but are nevertheless needed both at normal times and in particular during periods of developmental transition or stress. In maturity, selfobjects are perceived more realistically and less globally but, nevertheless, respond to and provide for our needs in circumstances when the self requires a temporary, though important, degree of support or uplifting.

Similarly, in analysis or therapy, according to Kohut, there is not in mature patients a decreasing interest in self needs over time, but the ability to identify and look after these oneself, or to turn for assistance when needed, is increased; the patient continues to expect that the therapist attend to his or her selfobject needs. If, however, a firm and secure self has not been attained and the self has floundered on the rocks of persistently inadequate selfobjects, the person will be less likely to deal with the tests of even normal misfortune, let alone exceptional ones. A person so handicapped may respond to such difficulties as though they constituted a grave injury or attack on the self and respond with rage and/or fragmentation. Kohut (Kohut and Wolf 1978) argues that a 'self-disorder' was defined as a structural propensity towards such break-ups and serious weakening of the self under stress.

We will dwell no longer on the wider theoretical background to Kohut's ideas, but the interested reader can consult Baker and Baker's 1987 review or the more critical discussions by Maratos (1988), Bacal (1995) and Mollon (1986).

### Narcissistic vulnerability

Although it would not be wise to apply a single diagnostic category to all addicted individuals, we suggest that what Kohut has formulated with respect to narcissistic personality disorder has most helpful implications for understanding addiction. Some of the phenomena that come to mind immediately from the clinical situation are low self-esteem, self-absorption, difficulties maintaining a balanced valuation of the self in relation to others (keeping a sense of proportion), an inability to soothe the self in a healthy fashion, when tensions arise, and other deficits in self-care. At least some of the relapses following sobriety seem significantly linked to anger, frustration and other felt threats to the self, during which the person resorts to previous solutions. The term 'narcissistic vulnerability', as I employ it here, can imply either a global weakness of the self, as hypothesised in narcissistic personality disorder proper, or can apply to more circumscribed areas of the personality in which the individual is particularly compromised, such as in feeling assertive or being able to socialise confidently.

In *The Analysis of the Self*, Kohut (1971) details how during the course of development we see a gradual building up of what he terms 'self-structures' – through a continual process of 'transmuting internalisation' – whereby the individual becomes less dependent on an actual object to perform the function of providing such structures. Self-structures allow the individual to begin to be able to arrive at and regulate his or her own wellbeing. Yet, in early periods of development, or at times of particular stress or transition, such structures are vulnerable and developmental attainments can be reversed or dismantled, throwing the individual back towards greater reliance on an external objects. Without self-structures which are sufficiently secured through experience and strengthened by the support of reliable selfobjects, no firm self is possible. Kohut argues in the latter case that the 'child does not acquire the needed internal structure, his psyche remains fixated on an archaic selfobject, and the person will throughout life be dependent on certain objects in what seems to be an intense form of object hunger' (1971, p. 46). Such individuals might present clinically as overtly needy, resourceless or aimlessly searching for something. These more archaic objects are not quite independent objects, seen in their own right, but are more primitive selfobjects whose role is to provide particular services or functions to the individual concerned.

### The drug as a selfobject

Perhaps, in drug addiction these early, archaic objects and object functions become realised in the inanimate form of substances or chemicals. Taking this view, the drug or the alcohol functions to the individual as a replacement selfobject. Kohut claims that that 'the drug, however, serves not as a substitute for loved or loving objects, or for a relation with them, but as a replacement for a defect in the psychological structure' (1971, p. 46). Artificial selfobjects like drugs may be sought in lieu of proper self-structures, and, in this case, there is no actual building of, or nutrients to, the self. The drug is seen as omnipotent, with the user able to conjure and recreate selfobject experiences, making it much more difficult to be able to learn from reality.

From the perspective of self-psychology, the drug acquires an alternative significance for dealing with life experience. The immediate manifestation of its use may be one or several of the following: an alteration in mood, a raising of self-esteem, an increased vitality or energy, a sense of power or assertion, an intense affective experience or a nullifying of intense experiences, taking the edge off reality. The immediacy of these effects – the short-term gain – offers a reassuring feeling of control or comfort. Temporarily, therefore, the taking in of the drug can lead to a feeling of triumph over problems within the self, but, however, this constitutes a pyrrhic victory.

Kohut describes how earlier, grandiose demands are relinquished throughout development, replaced hopefully by an acceptance of normal limitations, resulting in stable rather than labile self-esteem and, through the internalisation of idealised values, the person can sustain encouragement and enjoyment in the self and its achievements (1977a). Addicts, by contrast, appear enslaved by the drug (including the drug rituals and company) with a progressive weakening of other values or interests. The sustenance sought through drugs leads inevitably to further depletion of the individual's psychological resources and, in time, to demoralisation.

In *The Restoration of the Self*, Kohut (1977a) argues that the narcissistic disorders involve a serious defect in the self, acquired during childhood, and that defences or compensations are created to deal with these defects. Different forms of self-stimulation or addiction can substitute for growing up, providing false strength or a means of feeling alive and reassured. In his preface to a collection of papers on drug addiction, he goes further to claim that, 'By ingesting the drug he [the user] symbolically compels the mirroring selfobject to accept him. Or he symbolically compels the idealised selfobject to submit to his merging into it and thus to his partaking of its magical power' (1977b, p. vii). Tragically, the user disavows, either wholly or partially, his or her need for narcissistic sustenance from human selfobjects, turning instead to an inanimate selfobject that appears less likely to disappoint or refuse him or her.

### The malignant spiral of addiction

The following diagram (Figure 3.1) illustrates how some of Kohut's thinking could help clarify the nature of the vicious circle or spiral involved in addiction.

THE PROBLEM

A WORSE PROBLEM

There is a basic lack
of self-esteem or
cohesion, with
problems in self-
comforting or
initiation, leading to
a search elsewhere for
feelings of worth,
comfort and strength.

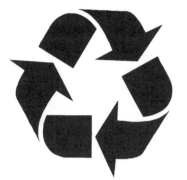

THE FLAW

Because this only
gives fleeting relief,
there is a need for
new supplies and
hence the need to
repeat the solution
over and over.

THE SOLUTION

Through the taking in of
the drug (or drink or
gamble) the user
manufactures the desired
feeling of being accepted,
stimulated or merged with
a source of power.
(Mirroring or idealising
needs.)

**Figure 3.1**: The self-defeating process.

Following this diagram through, we begin with an assumed weakness at the core of the personality, a defect in the self. This is recognised clinically in an abysmal sense of self-worth, in a poor self-soothing ability (that is to say an inability to maintain states of comfort and wellbeing) and in difficulties mobilising the self when assertion or self-protection are required. As for the latter, the addicts run many risks to themselves, traditionally explained in terms of self-destructive motives rather than as reflecting wider deficits in the self (see Khanztian 1990).

Moving further around the spiral of abuse, the various effects of the drugs once ingested provide for a short-lived, new self-state with the person locked into the prospect of an initial high or hit that might correspond to an artificially stimulated increase in self-esteem (either of the grandiose self or of attachment to the idealised object imago in Kohut's language). This is a mirage, a flawed solution and, 'as no psychic structure is built, the defect in the self remains' (Kohut 1977b, p. vii).

The search for external narcissistic supplies becomes an end in itself and over time results in the serious depletion and undermining of confidence. Caught in a malignant cycle, the person does not simply return to the beginning of the cycle but acquires each time round a new confirmation of not actually being able to resolve his or her central problems and so is in a yet worse predicament. In the diagram, this predicament is represented in terms of a spiral, with a chronic movement inwards or downwards. Such self-defeating mechanisms have been amply recognised in other approaches, like AA, in the form of helpful reminders or slogans, such as: 'We drank for joy and became miserable', 'We drank for strength and became weak', 'We drank for confidence and became doubtful' and so on.

There is some common ground between this view of addiction and other conceptualisations within the psychodynamic tradition, for example those of Rado (1933 1957) from a relatively more classical framework, or the more recent work of Wurmser (1978). Rado, for example, describes the way in which the drug comes to augment the ego and as a consequence distorts reality. When the reverse state sets in, following intoxication or the come down, he writes that, 'The ego is shrunken and reality appears exaggerated in its dimensions' (1933, p. 10); in his later paper he describes the drug's aftermath or withdrawal in the following manner: 'His situation is worse than before; he feels he must recapture yesterday's grandeur by taking another dose' (1957, p. 166). One might say that in both Kohut's and Rado's theories, there is in drug misuse an implied triumph of narcissism over experience, with devastating results for the capacity of the ego to learn from or to appraise reality.

Leon Wurmser (1978) hypothesises a 'cycle of addiction', which emphasises the centrality of what he calls 'narcissistic crises' as the precipitants of the cycle. Narcissistic crises involve some kind of serious disappointment or collapse in the view either of the grandiose self or of the idealised object. Some adolescents seem particularly vulnerable to such fluctuations. In his model, an individual's emotions regress, and aggression is mobilised; in the compulsive drug abuser, there is a consequent search for an 'affect defence' in the form of drugs to halt the further destabilisation of the personality. Unfortunately, the fact that the user buys only temporary relief of psychic pain – and is gratified in the short term – makes it more likely that the cycle of drug use is repeated.

### A note on narcissistic rage

In Shakespeare's *Antony and Cleopatra*, Cleopatra awaits news of her beloved who has had to return to Italy and where, for cynical and political reasons, he has married Octavia, the sister of the powerful Caesar. It will be recalled that Antony and Cleopatra's vision had been one of combined power and ultimate dominion through their relationship, and through the coming together of Rome and Egypt other kingdoms would be 'clay' in their hands. When the messenger returns to report to an anxious Cleopatra, she is barely able to allow him to talk and the messenger struggles nervously to bring to her, through instalments, the unpalatable reality of Antony's marriage. When he finally does so, she strikes and threatens him in an explosion of rage, in a fine example of the phenomenon of 'shooting the messenger'. Attempting to defend himself from the onslaught he calls out: 'Gracious madam / I that do bring the news made not the match' (Act 2, scene v). The messenger narrowly escapes the murderous wrath of Cleopatra, who then takes stock of the news.

Kohut (1972) differentiates anger and aggression from what he terms 'narcissistic rage'. Whereas the former has a more circumscribed and directed quality, arising, for example, out of a conflict in attaining some goal or desire, narcissistic rage is more global and the individual reacts as though his or her entire self is in danger. The individual who suffers such a threat to his or her self wants to destroy the source of the 'offence' and desperately re-establish control, like Cleopatra's violence when her worldview and fantasy are threatened. Kohut argues that the 'narcissistically vulnerable individual responds to actual – or anticipated – injury with flight or fight (narcissistic rage)' (1972, p. 379).

The propensity in addicts to a plummeting of self-confidence and self-cohesion under stress, may lead to primitive and destructive reactions of rage. If Kohut is right, the individual's narcissistic balance has been threatened and the ensuing crisis – which may involve tantrums, self-attack or other violence – is the chain reaction in a desperate attempt to regain control, restore honour and so on. It is interesting to dwell on the fact that some relapses, even after a considerable period of abstinence, may be triggered by perceived threats to the self – with uncontrollable feelings of frustration or deprivation in which the individual's resolve to change comes unstuck. In such relapses, perhaps, the drug use or alcohol binge is readily used as both a weapon and a defence, with someone or something else often blamed for having caused it (see Levin 1987 and Dodes 1990).

## Clinical issues

### (a) Individual treatment

The following clinical examples come from once-weekly psychotherapy with two substance misusers, a woman on a methadone prescription and a man in his first year of sobriety from alcohol.

*Sandy (late twenties)*

Sandy displayed acute narcissistic sensitivity with fears of being ignored, rejected and of not counting in the eyes of other people, including professionals. In fact, she elicited a dual response from professionals of (a) the wish to respond sympathetically, given her plaintive expression of helplessness and (b) subsequent discomfort at the bottomless nature of her demands – the more time given, the more she required. She acquired the tag 'manipulative' as well as 'needy'.

On starting psychotherapy, she sought constant reassurance regarding the arrangements for each appointment (though in reality this hardly changed), and this was understood and interpreted by the author (the therapist) as her feeling that I would drop her from my mind after each session – an example of her fear of not counting as well as an expectation of my lack of reliability. Her insecurity about treatment had a pervasive quality, calling forth the need for considerable patience and also enforced limits to the therapy (ending on time for example, which was an issue for her). There seemed to be a rapid activation of powerful narcissistic or selfobject transferences, including a wish for a perfect understanding of her needs, even without her having to put effort into expressing them.

Among the repeating themes as therapy proceeded was a preoccupation with my state of mind, involving the nature of my interest in her, my concentration, even on a minute-to-minute basis and a fear that she would incur not only my irritation but a degree of frustration that I would soon find unacceptable. In trying to understand these preoccupations – which, for long periods, it was possible only to try to describe and hold (for me as well as for Sandy) – I concluded that they all seemed to hinge on a profound narcissistic concern, both about herself and, through projection or expectation, about me. For instance, there was not only a fear that I would find something unacceptable about her and would want to terminate treatment but also a corresponding picture of me having a powerful narcissistic investment in myself and my views, and, if she contradicted this in any way, I would forcibly eject her from treatment. Among the narcissistic picture of me was the idea that I was proving myself as a therapist and that I needed to believe that my understanding would always be superior to her own – that *I* needed the treatment, *my* treatment, more than anything else, and certainly above her own needs. Also, could she really tolerate a situation in which someone was there to concentrate on her, or would this be too much and she would have to drop out? The need would become the fear, in the manner which is often recognised in the borderline patient who has a terror of driving the other person away.

One of the defences she adopted was of compliance (either from her to me or at other stages the expectation that I should comply with all of her requirements), which seemed partially related to early experiences of an emotionally underresponsive or non-mirroring mother and a father who seemed to tire easily of involvement with her and share little; in other words, a father who might not have been easy to experience as being strong or as being an alternative figure of idealisation. Drug and heroin abuse came onto the stage during adolescence and seemed to have supplied a feeling of being able to make an impact on the world and win recognition from her peer group: in other words, a feeling of self-cohesion and a means of raising self-esteem. Once in treatment, reductions in methadone (sometimes requested by Sandy and usually resisted when imposed by the clinic) led to enormous fears of being re-exposed to impotent and fragmenting feelings. Methadone, in addition to the physiological role it provided, played a role as a selfobject, possibly in Sandy's case to lessen rage and aggression. This was explored at some length in the therapy, the meanings around the provision of methadone.

As already indicated, a key dynamic in treatment with Sandy was her experience of me as a powerful and tyrannical figure, understood as a reactivation of an earlier traumatising selfobject (made more frightening by its confusion with her own tyrannical narcissistic needs). If frustrated in the course of 'my treatment', I would regard her as the cause of the offence and, as such, remove her: unceremoniously throw her out or, through a cleverly disguised pretext, get her discharged and blamed for the failure. Perhaps this was an illustration of how narcissistic rage fears can be powerfully projected onto the therapist, leading to further efforts by the patient to defend the self against possible retribution; the patient then feels they have to take flight or fight.

At the same time, in my countertransference, I experienced much difficulty with her tyrannical aspects and around the fact of her wish for perfect understanding on the one hand and her apparent lack of empathy towards others on the other. I gradually highlighted this in the relationship between us, including how she was well able to 'go for the jugular' when criticising me and the pattern of taking offence and expressing rage at my misunderstandings and oversights; this led her into a particular, predictable role as the injured party. The detailed exploration of such narcissistic deflations and rage reactions led to a shift in the transference with a relative lessening of her absolute fears towards me and a greater sense of the legitimacy of her own anger. The gradual interpretation of such patterns and the narcissistic fears underpinning them seemed to successfully contain Sandy and led to a better ability to discriminate feelings as well as an ability to better match 'punishment to the crime', so to speak, when misunderstandings did occur, with me or in her relationships outside. Anger could begin to replace indiscriminate rage and confusion.

It is difficult to convey in a brief vignette, just how complex were the processes of change and how tenuous the therapeutic alliance at different periods. During one such period, where there had been much suicidal ideation, Sandy commented that, in working with her, it must be like having to walk through a battle-scarred minefield. I think this was a measure of how much internal damage she had to contend with and the utter devastation that intravenous drug use had brought her, prior to treatment. In response, I said something rather like: 'I think it is very important for you to make sure that I know just how difficult your life and feelings are at the moment. It is like you have to fight off a terrible despondency inside you. But in talking about a minefield, I think you want me to know about the risks that I also face – maybe a fear that I will be a victim or a casualty as well.' Of course, there was much more dialogue, but I think the battleground imagery (which Sandy first brought in) is an excellent metaphor for being able to talk about the trail of devastation caused by drugs and about the depleted state the individuals find themselves in, once some kind of defeat has been accepted. Perhaps therapists act as a kind of hospital in such circumstances, addressing the patient's state and working with whatever wounds, whatever damage there may be; but they are also negotiators, trying to find the best possible terms of recovery, rebuilding confidence, reducing suspicions. They have, in addition, to help the patient to ward off any rearguard actions by the forces that would invite the person back into drug-taking.

Finally, for the purposes of this summary, the patient later developed (or expressed) the idea of being a special patient, perhaps with the idea of forming with me a bond of special understanding, possibly based on a deep longing for importance and a reaction against the fear of an object who might be unable to understand or reluctant to respond to her needs. A mirror transference seemed to oscillate with an idealising transference but led, over much time, to the building up of a less absolute, more independent need for a selfobject. Treatment came to have a less all-or-nothing, life-or-death connotation, though the seriousness of her addiction was acknowledged. No relapses to drugs took place, although she came close.

Sandy did make significant strides in building resilience (that is self-structures), being able to ask for attention in a more realistic manner and expecting a reasonable, though not perfect, response from others. There was less global anger or break-up in response to letdowns, with greater ability to discriminate different emotional states. Help in naming and discriminating different affective states had also been an aim throughout the therapy.

## Peter (early thirties)

Peter's early history involved his mother's alcoholism and the absence, through early abandonment, of a father. The quality of his mothering seemed to have been unreliable rather than universally poor, with better periods during which his mother was more in tune and responsive to his growing needs, though these would be lost abruptly when his mother returned to drinking. During longer periods of his mother's sobriety, there was some making up, and offers of material compensation. Peter had tried to please others, putting himself second – or nowhere – and giving the impression of having to be grateful for any acts of consideration shown to him. His self-esteem appeared tied to the degree to which he could help others with a corresponding disavowal of any right to his own feelings or views.

The task during the early stages of treatment centred around helping him to appreciate the moulding of his sense of self and worth around other people, based historically on his playing the parent or container to his own mother. She had needed him in many ways as her own exclusive selfobject, rather fulfilling the role of what McDougall (1986) has called the 'cork child', holding a needy parent together. This imagery may be particularly apposite when one is talking about a child's experience of a drinking parent. In the language of self-psychology, we might talk of bad or negative selfobjects. The approach in treatment was not one of conscious agreement with the patient as to how hard life had been or of any kind of direct reassurance (often a powerful temptation in the countertransference with deprived patients) but one of the careful elucidation of his unconscious needs. This led to a tremendously painful recognition of the legitimacy of his own basic narcissistic needs and his right to exist. The experience of rage through treatment was, indeed, an important attainment, but proved sufficiently containable not to have led to destabilisation or relapse.

In patients where the self has been at the mercy of an unreliable selfobject and where the parent has looked to the child as a source of or as an obstacle to his or her own narcissism, the child is likely to grow up overburdened, having little to be sure about concerning its own existence. Drugs can substitute a preferable feeling something over a feeling nothing, as appeared to have been the case with Peter's history of substance misuse. When it surfaced, the empty, vessel-like existence was intolerable. It also increased the intensity of the transference longings and Peter's difficulty in imagining he could be an important and well-regarded individual in my mind.

With patients like Sandy and Peter, but perhaps with most addicts, one hopes to help the individual to rebuild or to acquire what Kohut might have phrased as being suitable 'endopsychic resources or structures'.

## (b) Supervision

The following vignettes derive from the supervision of psychiatric nurses, who were the mainstay of counselling and psychosocial support in the substance-misuse service in which I was based. I suggest that Kohut's ideas can assist the supervisor in appreciating the selfobject needs of the supervisee, and how these might interact with and confuse the different selfobject needs of the patient; recognition of these professional/personal needs can reduce confusion, freeing up the ability to learn new things with and from our patients.

### (i) 'Needing to be needed'

A drug worker with a strong identification with being helpful tended to react slightly depressively after seeing patients a few times, particularly after some initial sense of promise (evoked in part by the patient and in part by what the healthcare professional wanted to see) had worn off. With one patient, whom she regarded as having much potential behind a self-defeating façade, she became enthusiastically engaged in response to patient's periodic reports of promising developments in outside life: jobs, relationships and so on. However, the patient's depressed and lethargic side was strong and would sweep over her plans, paved with good intentions, and stimulant drugs provided a boost followed by further stagnation and disinterest. As the counselling unfolded, the healthcare professional's enthusiasm wore off, and her moods seemed increasingly to mirror those of the patient – engagement and disengagement, enthusiasm and depression – following in a less extreme manner the ups and downs of the patient's self-esteem.

Some of the patient's material then began to suggest an unconscious recognition of this process in the relationship between them, leading to an effort to keep the nurse interested and rewarded, as though the patient had internalised a now-demoralised healthcare professional on top of her own problems! Later on, however, the patient started to miss appointments and act out in other ways. The healthcare professional found it hard to empathise with these self-defeating cycles in this patient – seemingly unable to apply her preferred philosophy of positive thinking – and tended to shift her interest unknowingly to her new cases, in the same way she had done with this patient earlier. Of course, the process was subtle, but there was something about the nurse's tone of reporting that, with some exploration, led into particular underlying schemas of expectation of what a good client should be like.

In supervision, this was then developed in terms of the healthcare professional's difficulty in learning about the chronic nature of addiction – the malignant cycle of abuse – and how there had come to be a mix-up between the patient's needs and the worker's own investments. The healthcare professional was able to start to listen more carefully and cautiously to the patient. I believe that, for the supervisor to be helpful, the professional's own experience of their clients and their own narcissistic needs (for example to be seen as being helpful, to be seen in a good light and so on) have to be contained in some way. From this, more reflective counselling can proceed.

### (ii) 'On my level'

A nurse had chosen to work with drug addicts as she felt affinity with younger people and thought she could understand the culture of drug-taking. There was, on getting to know her better, a wish to be idealised by her patients and a conviction of being able to be on the same level as the younger patients. On the other hand, she did not want to be seen as a push over, adopting the philosophy that respect will beget respect, in a benign cycle of trust. The nurse frequently used the word 'trust' in her clinical reports.

During the course of work with one patient, the nurse found herself strongly identified with the patient in a particular difference in under-standing involving the patient and another professional – openly expressing her agreement with her patient – and gravitated towards being the patient's champion in the clinical discussions. Like the patient, the staff member tended to see the service system as being unfair. The client felt the nurse was the only person who supported her. Subsequently, some important facts were discovered, shifting the nurse's sympathy towards the other professional involved, and she felt let down by the patient. The nurse found it hard to begin to think about the contribution of a cynical selfobject in the patient's mind (which I think was based, historically, on a cynical and highly cruel father), which was usually projected outwards so that the world would be seen as unjust. Subsequently, the nurse was barely able to contain her own anger towards the patient, part of which stemmed from the patient's emotional switching to an attitude of devalu-ation towards the nurse. The patient no longer idealised the nurse, and the nurse's principle of respect (partly based on an overidentification with the patient's belief that she had been wronged by life in some way) had not turned the patient round, as expected.

In supervision, it was suggested that this cynical aspect of the patient was linked in her history to an identification with her father as an aggressor and with his particular techniques of devaluation towards her. One of the traps of a patient like this, particularly when there is an appealing side to the patient, is to fall into the unconscious agreement of: 'You and me against the outside world' (see Imhoff et al 1983). In terms of the nurse's awareness, she became more able to see her own need for a particular type of 'good' patient, and how there had indeed been a fall from grace in this case – the nurse's own narcissism and guiding principles had been wounded.

## Countertransference: a self-psychology orientation

In line with other psychoanalytic approaches, the countertransference reactions of the therapist are regarded as providing important elements of information about the patient, but also give clues as to the sensitivities and propensities of the professional engaged in the work. As is hopefully already clear from the supervision examples cited, major problems can and do arise from the interaction between the patient's narcissism – or intense selfobject needs – and the personal or professional narcissism of the therapist. No doubt particular constellations of transference and countertransference arise with addicted individuals, and it must be stressed here that an understanding of this area will be of relevance not only to in-depth psychotherapy but also to counselling and general psychosocial support. The following list is intended as a possible, not exhaustive, range of the problems involved, influenced by a self-psychology perspective. In each case I have given a simple heading to describe what might be depicted as the professional's starting point.

## The wish to be able to understand

Patients with addiction often demonstrate a counterdependent attitude to the treatment, as though they are saying that all their needs have already been taken care of through the drugs. This physical tie to the drug and corresponding inability to turn to a human figure can be difficult for the healthcare professional, who may feel overlooked or treated as secondary, to comprehend. This may be further complicated in clinics that prescribe substitute medication, like methadone. The professional may experience an equivalent of the spouse's or relative's exasperated experience of not being able to understand the addiction or even an equivalent to: 'It is either me or the drugs!' Unfortunately, the healthcare professional can play into this process by keeping the patient at arm's length, which cuts short the task of understanding the patient and allows us to put the patient out of our minds.

## The need to feel effective

Drugs, as we have speculated, act as the preferred selfobject to the user. While similar to our first heading, I am particularly emphasising the individual's reliance on an impersonal or inanimate container. The professional's sense of efficacy and his or her ability to influence others through *human* contact and understanding can be severely challenged by this. Once again, too much emphasis on the medical side of management can serve as a defence against experiencing the many difficulties and time involved in forging a therapeutic relationship with substance misusers.

## The wish to be helpful

Though not exclusive to the addicted patients, we are frequently devalued in our efforts and subject to the complaint that we have got it all wrong. Patients who devalue can challenge the professional's defences and resilience severely. Devaluations probably impede empathy or the wish to be empathic more often than most other transferences – because of the kind of abuse of a relationship that is implied – and need a good degree of self-observation, confidence and often the help of a third party for them to be recognised and contained in a therapeutic manner. The professional's identification with being helpful is likely to feel threatened and so the professional becomes the defensive one.

## To be respected: to have one's integrity recognised

Related to the foregoing theme, the professional may be on the receiving end of periodic or sustained attacks on his or her perceived values, and often the patients will try to identify a sensitive area of the worker's professional (if not personal) identity: a doctor who is not doing his or her job properly, a nurse who does not care, a social worker who leaves them empty-handed or a psychotherapist who does not understand them would be examples. Other patients may express this attack through a theme of corruption and mistrust of authority, which can leave even the experienced therapist or doctor shaken and defensive. Some healthcare professionals are tempted in circumstances like these to reassert their own position, sometimes rationalised in terms of confronting the patient.

In terms of handling mirror transferences, considerable countertransference strains can arise in response to the patient who can only see their own needs and is expectant of perfect understanding, as with the treatment of Sandy described above. For long periods – with or without accurate understanding – the patient can remain fixated on his or her grandiose self and may, as Kohut (1977a) argues, experience the therapist as a threat to this or as a foreign body; some patients will be unable to tolerate the idea that someone else might have a different picture from how they see themselves, as this will be a narcissistic threat. In some forms of mirror transference, such as 'merging' or 'twinship', the therapist may not be seen as an individual at all, carrying for the patient a more impersonal containing function. Such blotting out of the therapist can be intolerable for the professional to experience if their sense of their own significance as a person is sufficiently undermined. The therapist has to manage many role reductions of this kind and may feel outraged when on the receiving end of a selfobject need in the patient.(See Bacal's 1995 discussion.)

### The wish for a realistic relationship

As for the idealising transferences, some therapists feel uncomfortable with being idealised at all by the patient, if this affronts their more egalitarian preferences, while other therapists may, on being idealised, feel stimulated in their own grandiosity and start to overestimate their powers. More difficult to attain, perhaps, is an optimal degree of acceptance of a patient's idealisation and a resilience in the face of subsequent belittlement when we fail to live up to the patient's omnipotent wishes.

### The wish to make better

Finally, we must not forget that many of our patients will have suffered sometimes enormous, actual deprivation in which damaged and unmet narcissistic needs will be an important feature. Basic needs may not have been mirrored or responded to reliably, with the person further handicapped by the rejections of other, potentially idealiseable selfobjects that might have otherwise supplied some measure of compensation. While the drugs may have given the user the illusion of now being free from his or her past, they actually make him or her even less available to be helped in the present. Rescue fantasies can arise in the professional, and mirroring can be misused to imply a kindly, oversympathetic response. Perhaps the therapist starts to offer more than he or she can deliver. This is dangerous when not identified, as Goldberg (1980) suggests. There may be the hidden wish with deprived patients 'to supply in the here and now for the deprivation of the past'(p. 423).

## Conclusion

Kohut's work, and that of others who have extended self-psychology, offers an illuminating perspective on addiction and its treatment, which can be summarised thus:

1. It orientates us to areas of narcissistic vulnerability and self-defects in the patients whom we see, as well as the extreme defences against such problems.
2. We are helped to understand the propensity to rage and aggression often encountered (due to threats to the self), with the user turning to substances as a contradictory measure to reassert control for the purposes of survival. This may reflect the patient's chronic sense of powerlessness.
3. The supervisor and the professional can think more sensitively about the interaction between their own needs/vulnerabilities and those of the patient. This can enhance empathy and responsiveness.

Some qualifications are also needed.

Kohut treated patients with predominantly narcissistic personality disorder. By contrast, there is no general personality type for addicted individuals, though the wider notion of damage to and deficits of the self is one which can be applied to different personalities and temperaments. It is a structural concept.

Some individuals have extensive damage to the self, long before an addiction is acquired. The addiction offers false sustenance or structure. On the other hand, narcissistic vulnerability is also a consequence of the addiction, as self-structures are eroded. In many cases, there will be a tragic interaction between the two, expressed in the idea of the malignant spiral. Self-psychology should not be thought of as offering a simple choice between, or polarity of, 'cause' and 'consequence' in addiction.

Finally, I would add that the ideas here do not imply that all substance misusers should receive self-psychological psychotherapy or analysis, quite the contrary. Substance misusers require a wide range of treatments in both individual, familial and group modalities. However, the contribution of self-psychological ideas can be helpful, even in non-analytic therapy, as a framework of understanding. Different clinical approaches that are responsive to the particular sensitivities of our clients can go a long way in facilitating change and in ameliorating isolation and other character defences in addicted individuals.

# Part 2
# Therapy

# CHAPTER 4
# The dynamics of addiction in the clinical situation

## ROBERT COHEN

Patients with addiction problems are not popular with medical or psychiatric staff, who are often puzzled and distressed by the patients' behaviour. Addicted patients, whatever their drug of choice, do not interact in the same way as other patients for reasons that can be explained by the psychodynamics of addiction. This often leads to interactions that are not helpful to the patient or the staff, with frequently undesirable outcomes. However, if the dynamics of the situation are understood, strategies can be devised to handle situations to lead to a more favourable outcome. This chapter aims to highlight some of the more frequently observed dynamics and make suggestions about how they might be handled. It is not intended to advocate the introduction of further psychological therapies (not that they are not needed) but to indicate that attention to psychodynamic factors *in the routine clinical situation* (where time-consuming interventions such as interpretation of the transference, as occurs in formal psychoanalytical settings, are not practicable) can suggest practical steps that will assist the therapist in handling the clinical encounter more satisfactorily for both the therapist and the patient. The suggestions in this chapter are relevant to the management of addicted patients in general medical and paramedical settings, in hospital and in general practice, as well as in the more specialised setting of the psychiatric clinic and the drug dependence unit.

Studies of the natural history of addiction show that it is a disorder that develops over a long period of time and that recovery, when it occurs, follows a protracted and fragile course. Aetiological studies do not reveal causes of addiction but predisposing factors – examples include the genetically determined flushing reaction to alcohol typical of Oriental people that reduces the likelihood of the development of subsequent alcoholism and the increased frequency of histories of physical and/or sexual abuse in

53

the childhoods of patients who subsequently become addicted (although increased frequency of either forms of abuse predisposes to an increased likelihood of a number of psychiatric disorders).

However, observers of addicted patients will notice a number of psychological and psychodynamic features in patients who are at the early stages of seeking treatment, when they may appear unmotivated and resistant to change, such as avoidance of responsibility, hostility and inter-personal difficulties that change with the development of recovery from addiction into self-efficacy, taking responsibility and interacting with others in a more appropriate and effective way. The patient in denial displays the features of a failure to cope with the demands that life presents (when the psychoactive drug is used as an alternative, simple – but entirely ineffective – solution to life problems), with recovery involving the development of these mechanisms that occur in most other people as the transition from adolescence to adulthood is successfully negotiated. Indeed, the current author would suggest that addiction to any psychoactive drug (including tobacco) is primarily a variant of a psychological disorder in which the person either fails to develop adult psychological mechanisms of self-efficacy (primary addiction) or when under great stress regresses to use of the psychological mechanisms that are appropriate in childhood (secondary addiction). In addiction to a psychoactive substance, the drug is being substituted for more sophisti-cated, adult mechanisms of behaving.

## Developmental changes

To clarify this argument that addiction is a disorder of psychological devel-opment, a schematic representation of developmental changes in psychology over time is presented here. Human beings have developed to have a prolonged childhood in which the child is looked after by the parent.

### The newborn child

At birth, the newborn child is entirely dependent on its parents (usually mother) or other carer to meet its needs for food, warmth, affection and bodily toilet. Having not yet acquired a number of skills, such as speech, locomotion and fine grasp, the infant can neither obtain directly nor communicate clearly to its parent what is needs or wants at the time. The child can only communicate non-verbally with a cry, and it cannot directly enforce its carer to do its bidding. Thus, the child *has* to rely on the carer to interpret what its needs are for it and can only use manipulative techniques to ensure that the parent will attend to it. A psychological manipulation is a request coupled with a contingency, and, while the cry alerts the parent to the fact that it requires something, it is the piercing nature of the cry that persuades a reluctant parent to attend directly. Thus, it may be the middle of the night and she might be exhausted, having fed the child only one hour ago, but the mother will still put the child to the breast if only to shut the child up! And the child will call at any time of night or day – there is no delay between the baby needing something and crying.

Thus, the baby shows non-verbal communication, manipulative behaviour, dependence on another (with expectation that the other will think for it), absence of delay for gratification and external locus of control. A baby whose needs are not met despite its unclear behaviour becomes irritable and angry. There is no respect for the needs of the mother.

### The growing child

As the child grows, it gradually develops all these skills that it lacked as a baby. It learns to communicate verbally, whereby it can learn to make choices, obtain what it needs for itself directly (getting food out of a cupboard, see to its own toileting, put on an extra jumper, make its own friends) or otherwise, where help is required, indicate what those choices are and respect the needs of the other enough to tolerate delayed gratification. In this way, the growing child obtains mastery over the world and can develop an internal locus of control, the ability to make a direct request as well as manipulation (or force, which it may now have), the ability to tolerate delayed gratification and the ability to satisfy its needs.

For some, however, this process is interrupted or fails. Inconsistent parenting may mean that a child does not learn how successful a direct request can be but instead discovers the efficacy of an indirect (manipulative) one. If the child does not receive what it needs even after a delay, it does not learn that there is any point waiting, and the ability to tolerate delayed gratification does not occur. If no adult spends much time with the child, verbal skills are developed much less. A repeated series of failures leads the child to feel that it has no mastery over the world. It fails to make choices, and this reinforces the cycle of feeling that there is no choice or that things are out of control. The child constantly feels miserable for failing and angry at the unwillingness of those close to it to provide it with what it needs. It does not develop a sense of value. If there has been frequent physical or sexual abuse, even the child's own body is not safe nor unavailable to others – that is the boundary between the child and others' bodies is not clearly marked.

## The adolescent

After ten or fifteen years of this, it is not surprising when a simple solution is suggested it is considered. Take a drug and you will feel better. To the adolescent's surprise, it does. The move from insecure attachment to a parental figure to an insecure attachment (albeit less so) to a psychoactive substance is an easy step.

## Staff and patients

When the patient then presents at a service for the treatment of an addiction (to alcohol, opiates, stimulants, benzodiazepine, cannabis, other drug or a combination of these), the staff see the body of an adult. They may not understand that some of the mental processes are still those of a child. In addition, the staff in the helping professions are often there because of their own dependency needs, and, as well as failing to realise that expectations of adult behaviour in the addict are unrealistic, they may be less able to tolerate the demanding behaviours of the patient. There is a recipe for inappropriate behaviours on the part of both patient and staff member, leading to inappropriate and sometimes harmful therapy.

The problems of the countertransference induced in the staff member are discussed elsewhere in this book. In this chapter, the focus will be on the dynamics of the patient and some practical measures that the staff member can take to improve the likelihood of managing a clinical encounter appropriately.

On the basis of this schema, a description of the dynamics of the unrecovered addict would include a narcissistic and manipulative individual with poor self-esteem and self-efficacy with an external locus of control and one who is prone to splitting, breaking boundaries, magical thinking, avoidant behaviour and acting out. Table 4.1 lists these and the differences noted in recovered addicts (these are also present in mature, non-addicted individuals). In both normal psychological development and recovery from addiction, mature mechanisms are added to previous immature mechanisms but do not replace them. At times of stress, a reversion to use of more immature features can occur. This would account, psychodynamically, for the situation of an addicted patient who relapses after many years of abstinence or the development of an addiction in a previously normal person who undergoes great stress. (The present author has seen patients who have developed addiction to opiates used for the treatment of metastatic cancer and patients who have developed addiction to opiates and benzodiazepines as a grief response to terminal illness such as the final stages of AIDS.)

**Table 4.1:** Features of dynamics of addiction

| Unrecovered addict | | Addict in recovery |
|---|---|---|
| External locus of control | ↔ | Internal locus of control |
| Irresponsible | ↔ | Takes responsibility |
| Poor self-esteem | ↔ | Satisfactory self-esteem |
| Ambivalence | ↔ | Clear decision-making |
| Magical thinking | ↔ | Realistic thinking |
| Manipulative behaviour | ↔ | Direct request |
| Avoidance/denial | ↔ | Acceptance of reality |
| Narcissism | ↔ | Altruism |
| Splitting | ↔ | Integration |
| Boundary-breaking | ↔ | Respecting boundaries |
| Withdrawal/escape | ↔ | Facing up to problems/conflict/feelings |
| Repression | ↔ | Suppression/sublimation |
| Acting out | ↔ | Able to contain own feelings |

This table shows in the left-hand column the dynamics that addicts show while they are still using drugs, in the right-hand column, the new dynamics that the addicts use when they have ceased using drugs because they are in recovery from the disorder.

## Self-esteem and control

The main areas of difficulty for the addicted person relate to self-esteem and control (both of which are very low) in the context of a narcissistic personality structure, in which either there is an absence of recognition of others as people rather than objects or the boundaries between the individual and others are very indistinct. While this situation may be advantageous in an infant, it makes it hard for an older person to avoid distressing situations arising. The processes of psychological maturation which involve the addition of mechanisms that allow the person to contain his or her own anxiety (such as sublimation and rationalisation) do not develop adequately in addicted people and so mechanisms of dealing with distress involve avoidance (denial or repression) or externalisation (projection, reaction-formation or identification with the aggressor) leading to the person ceding control and hierarchical superiority (and with it greater self-esteem) to another. Although the immediate effect is to reduce psychological distress, the cost is reinforcement of low self-esteem and low control, thus creating a vicious circle. For the addict, the drug can act as an object no less than a person: the drug can be an object of avoidance or externalisation. Assisting the addict in the long term requires support of the development of appropriate control and appropriate self-esteem.

In the clinical situation, addicted patients show an intense selfishness with little respect to the therapist. They do not take responsibility for their actions, preferring to depend on the therapist, whose own needs may be made secondary to the patient's immediate need for gratification. The therapist experiences a demanding, unsatisfied, possibly angry, hostile or critical patient who frequently tries to break boundaries (using inappropriate control techniques). The therapist thus experiences an attack on his or her own self-esteem and power of control; it is this attack (especially if perceived by the therapist as successful in the patient's terms) that causes distress in the therapist. The inexperienced therapist may respond by attempting to gratify the patient (for example by supplying a higher dose of an opiate drug, thus reinforcing the maladaptive patient dynamic or by rejecting the patient). Both these responses involve the therapist using the same immature maladaptive dynamic as the patient (that is, identification or denial), thereby colluding with the patient maintaining his or her own maladaptive psycho-dynamic status quo.

Table 4.2 lists some of the dynamics operating in addicted patients. It should be borne in mind that not all patients show all these dynamics all of the time, but the staff member should be aware that they might become manifest. The various dynamics arising both out of the narcissistic person-ality structure and from the immature defence mechanisms are not isolated and may interact.

The resultant behaviours are therefore complex, and different combi-nations may lead to diametrically opposite behaviour. For example, an addict may refuse to attempt to detoxify from the substance(s) of choice because the problem is one of supply, not a recognition that there is a problem; conversely, a patient may insist on attempting to detoxify even when not ready (for example because there is a recognition of a problem, but detoxification is seen as an easy solution, and the patient focuses on detoxification *instead* of recovery, not as a first step in recovery). Alternatively, the same example illustrates that the same behaviours for example attempting detoxification, can be a sign of improvement in one patient while a sign of denial in another. It is the experienced therapist who can determine which dynamic is acting and whether a proposed course of action is likely to be helpful or unhelpful to the patient.

### The narcissistic patient

The narcissistic patient is unable to recognise the reality of other people. The person perceives that the world centres around them and other people are there for the benefit of that person. The patient indicates this with talk that is self-centred. For example, many patients on opiate or benzodiazepine-substitution therapy talk of 'my script'. While this may

Table 4.2: How the unrecovered addict manifests addictive pathology

| Psychoanalytic element | Cognitive psychological element | Interacting dynamic | Modality | Interacting dynamic | Practical example |
|---|---|---|---|---|---|
| *Features of immature and fractured ego* | | | | | |
| narcissism | selfishness | | speech | | where is my script? |
| | | | action | | attends late for appointment |
| | | | | boundary breaking | see text |
| | | | | projection and external locus of control | boredom (another responsible for his/her entertainment), unemployment |
| | | | | | interactive style instrumental |
| splitting | | | | | see text |
| poor self-containment | labile emotions | | speech | | easily becomes angry, anxious, happy |
| | | | speech | | inability to tolerate delayed gratification |
| | | | action | | acting out, sadistic/masochistic use of drug |

(Continues)

Table 4.2: Continued

| Psychoanalytic element | Cognitive psychological element | Interacting dynamic | Modality | Interacting dynamic | Practical example |
|---|---|---|---|---|---|
| *Immature psychological defence mechanisms* | | | | | |
| projection | external locus of control | | speech | | 'What do you want me to do, doctor?' |
| | | | action | | comes for treatment to avoid a prison sentence/loss of a partner |
| | | reaction formation | action | impotence | over controlling behaviour – threats, anger, violence, hostage taking |
| | | low self-esteem | speech | guilt, shame | |
| | | | action | | |
| | | low self-esteem and reaction formation | speech | grandiosity, sarcasm, contempt, putting the other down | |
| | | low self-efficacy | action | | |

| mechanism | speech/action | example |
|---|---|---|
| low self-efficacy and magical thinking | action | dependence on therapist; expectation that a person will solve all problems (e.g. a new lover), just as the drug should |
| denial | speech | 'I only drink socially' |
| projection | speech | 'Don't tell me that I drink too much, doctor' |
| | speech | tells lies (self-deceit) |
| | action | fails to attend an appointment |
| avoidance/escape | speech | 'I'm not going to talk about that now' |
| | action | gets drunk to escape an argument |
| magical thinking | speech | 'I will not relapse, through willpower' |
| fantasy/unrealistic expectation | action | goes to pub, expecting not to be tempted to drink (set up) |

appear no more than a convenient shorthand, it is often a statement of ownership – the patient comes to think of the medication as something that he or she owns and to which he or she has an entitlement. But a prescription is a recommendation by a medical practitioner of treatment. In taking the prescription as a right, many patients behave as though the doctor no longer has any right to determine the dose, frequency of administration, frequency of dispensing or duration of treatment. If a doctor then decides that the treatment is not working and that it should be terminated, the patient sees this not as a piece of medical advice but as the doctor depriving the patient of their property. When the doctor does try to assert himself or herself, much distress arises, as the patient believes he or she has a right to feel aggrieved. The additional dynamic in this situation is that the patient determines the medical treatment while the doctor prescribing takes responsibility. The patient in this situation believes he or she has control of the benefits of taking the drug, but, if anything goes wrong, the prescriber can always be blamed (covert externalisation). Many clinic staff collude with the narcissistic dynamic of the patient in respect of medication, believing erroneously that they have to be the advocate of the patient to a doctor who may have been employed in an emasculated capacity as a prescribing doctor. The effective way to deal with this (having recognised the dynamic) is to treat the interaction between patient and prescriber as involving two people. The patient is seeking advice, and the prescriber is offering what they believe to be of benefit to the patient, not necessarily what the patient wishes to hear.

There is room for a frank exchange of views, but the person taking responsibility for the medication has the right to have the final word in what he or she will write. If the patient desires a supply of the drug, in a manner different to that advised by the doctor, the patient will have to take responsibility for the supply. In practice, this means obtaining drugs from the street, but, if a patient cannot agree with the doctor about treatment, there is no reason to believe that the patient will not obtain drugs from the street anyway. It is therefore reasonable for a clinic to maintain that it has the final say about prescribed medication, and this should be made clear to all patients at the outset of treatment.

Patients will show their lack of awareness of others in their actions, as well as their words. Many patients will be late for appointments. For some, this is an attempt to reduce the possibility of interaction with staff beyond obtaining a prescription (that is, to avoid counselling, and in this way to avoid looking at their addiction). For others, it is simply that as the world appears to revolve around them; the needs of others are irrelevant – this patient expects people to be available at any time that it suits them, and, if it suits the patient to turn up late, then (the patient thinks), why not? But social interaction requires an awareness of the pressures on others, and if the patient attends at a time different from the appointment, the staff member may be otherwise occupied. The patient may have lost jobs and other societal benefits on other occasions when he or she has not arrived on time. It is therefore important for the clinic to insist on punctuality, and the patient who is late should not be seen. The lesson does require that the staff members show the same respect to the patient, and staff members should make the most strenuous effort not to be late for the appointment.

In describing these interactions, many readers might be tempted to regard matters such as close attention to punctuality as petty. Such readers would be misguided, as it is these apparently trivial matters that are the core of addiction (and its treatment) and the very matters that are overlooked that make understanding of the addictive process so difficult.

The reader might also be tempted to regard the description of the behaviour of the staff as an attempt to control patients or demonstrate superiority. Such readers would be misreading the paragraphs; in the case of the prescription, the attempt is not that one member of the encounter, either the patient or the doctor, should be dominant, but that there should be an equality – with the possibility that at the end of the interview it should be acceptable that the two parties have different opinions. It is this lack of recognition of the importance of *equality* in the interaction that has hindered the development of effective drug services.

## Interpersonal boundaries

The lack of awareness of others as separate individuals leads to difficulties with interpersonal boundaries. Patients may attempt to contact the staff member at home or outside of hours, may try to treat the staff member as a friend rather than as a professional adviser, may ask for the staff member to join in social activities with him or her, may ask for a sexual relationship and may attempt a number of other intrusions that are inappropriate. The staff member can deal with this by reminding the patient in word and deed that this is a formal relationship, not an intimate one, and that interactions should be limited to what is required in the therapeutic setting. In the current climate of addressing people by their first names, staff should nevertheless consider the use of titles – a doctor who insists on being called 'Dr X' and not by his or her first name is constantly and appropriately reminding the patient that the relationship is entirely professional, not social. In accordance with the importance of maintaining equality in the relationship, the doctor who rightly insists on the use of his or her title should similarly address the patient as 'Mr/Mrs Y' and not by his or her first name either. This needs to be handled delicately, as many addicted patients do not expect to be addressed by a title, but, as well as equality, this is a non-verbal way of enhancing the patient's esteem.

The patient (possibly for the first time in his or her life) is being treated as a real adult. Similarly, the staff member should make a point of seeing the patient only in the healthcare setting. On the rare occasions that a home visit is *clinically* appropriate, normal procedures for home visiting should be applied, including professionals visiting in pairs, at a designated time for a designated purpose. Conversations in therapeutic sessions should be limited to matters relating to the treatment of the addiction; there is no need for the staff member to disclose personal details (to an addict, these are not of real interest but can serve as weapons against the staff member in the future and a spurious basis for the patient avoiding taking required action, for example it is not relevant whether the staff member is an addict in recovery or not). Social and sexual relations with patients are entirely inappropriate at all times.

In the narcissistic state, the patient learns that giving is sometimes necessary for receiving (for example giving money to a dealer to get drugs) but does not learn to do things for others for nothing in return. Thus inter-actions are usually instrumental rather than altruistic. If the patient believes that they are giving something, they will expect something in return. For example, if a patient attends on time at the insistence of the clinic staff, he or she will expect something in return (it might be that they have an increase in their script in mind). This should be anticipated as, if not understood, a staff member might be surprised at the emotional display, often of anger, of the patient who is not gratified in the way he or she expects. The staff member can deal with this in the long term by clari-fying that certain matters (for example punctuality) are not concessions made for the *staff* by the patient, but rather requirements and responsibil-ities of the patient to *him- or herself*.

## Ambivalence

One of the hardest aspects of treating addicts is the feature of *ambiva-lence*. The origin of this psychodynamic feature is that the ego has not become integrated. According to Klein (1957), the patient has not success-fully made the transition from the paranoid-schizoid to the depressive position. In practice, this means that the patient sees things in black and white and will divide people and things off into good and bad. He or she will play one professional off against another. For example, he or she may behave as though the DDU doctor is bad and the GP is good (or vice versa). When the DDU doctor refuses the patient's request (for example to increase the dose of the prescription) confirming in the patient's mind that the doctor is bad, the patient will approach the GP. The message to the GP will be that the GP is good, unlike the bad DDU doctor. The undeclared threat to the GP is that if they wish to maintain their position as good doctor, they should do the patient's bidding. An unwary professional in the good position may well indulge the patient. Although in this example, two doctors have been used, any two (or more) professionals can be split in this way. When the two professionals come from different disciplines, perhaps with different treatment philosophies, there is a risk of very severe damage being done if the splitting of the patient is not dealt with appropriately. Nor is it difficult to manage.

The mechanism often involves the patient *reporting* the words of one professional to another ('Dr Bloggs said that you would do such and such for me'; 'Mr Bloggs, social worker, doesn't understand that I need such and such'). These statements by the patient may be true, but they may also be only partially true or even false. The professional hearing them would be wise to inquire of the first professional what was said and meant, rather than acting on the word of the client (especially if the second professional finds his or her emotions aroused against the first professional by the report of the patient). The summary of this is that professionals involved in the treatment of patients are wise to communicate directly, rather than indirectly via patients (even inadvertently).

Professionals are also advised to guard against splitting by addicts by having one person as the centre of all communications – that is, a keyworker. That person should co-ordinate the current plan of treatment, and other involved professionals should seek the current state of play from the keyworker directly before making decisions about addiction treatment. It is the advice of the current author that such a keyworker should be in secondary care (that is in a DDU) and not primary care (general medical practice) where expertise is limited. Resources are deficient in both primary and secondary care in the UK for the treatment of addicts and should be resolved by increasing the resources available in secondary care, not by insisting that a clinically inappropriate course be undertaken as it is seen as cheaper.

The *ambivalence* of the patient arising out of the lack of ego-integration often confuses clinicians and is often misinterpreted. Ambivalence is shown in more than one way. It is shown by the patient saying that they want something (for example the goal of abstinence) and its opposite (for example to continue to use a little) at the same time (that is, the patient wants to have their cake and eat it) or by the patient who wants to pursue a course of action (for example go to residential rehabili-tation) but cannot make up their mind about which centre they will apply to. The result in the first example is that the patient continues to use and in the second that the patient does not attend rehabilitation as he or she does not decide. In other words, the ambivalence of the patient prevents any change occurring.

It is important that the clinician realises that the patient is not feigning, and that failure to make decisions is not necessarily malicious nor intended as a deception. Belief on the part of the clinician that the ambivalent patient is lying or deceiving may lead the clinician to think less well of the patient, and the resultant deterioration of the relationship will be clinically harmful. The clinician can handle the situation by recognising the ambivalence and allowing the patient to think about it. In the case of the patient who is ambivalent about whether to give up using drugs, the clinician can assist by spending time discussing whether the patient does really wish to give up at the present time. In the case of a choice, the clinician can assist the patient by forcing a choice. For example, a clinician may agree to arrange for detoxification only when the patient has chosen (and applied to) a rehabilitation centre to which he or she will go immediately after detoxification.

The patient may make the choice that the clinician does not agree with (for example to continue to use), but the right to make such choices (and have them respected) should be left entirely with the patient – who has to bear the consequences. An alcohol-dependent patient with medical evidence of extensive liver damage has the right to decide to continue to drink, as he or she will be the one to die when the liver is finally destroyed. Similarly, an opiate-dependent patient who continues to use cocaine on top of his or her methadone script has the right to decide to continue to do so, but he or she should not be spared the consequence of being discharged from treatment if the use of cocaine on top is forbidden as part of the treatment contract. The change from thinking that you can have your cake and eat it (splitting) to thinking that actions have consequences is an important cognitive *and* psychodynamic change on the road to recovery from addiction.

**Containment of emotions**

The difficulty with boundaries, resulting from the inability to distinguish between the self and others, also manifests itself in a difficulty in containment of a patient's own emotions, thoughts and actions. Responses of anger, laughter or tears come quickly when provoked. When the patient requests something, he or she finds it very hard to wait if not given it immediately (difficulty in tolerating delayed gratification) and becomes quickly irritable, complaining and persistent. The clinic staff member may respond by trying to deal with the patient's demand immediately, even if in the middle of doing something else, or, conversely, the staff member may become angry in response to the persistent nature of the demand and deliberately make the patient wait more than otherwise. Both these responses are inappropriate. Rather, the staff member should try to behave with the patient as he or she would with any other adult, both as a practical step and as a learning experience for the patient. As with anyone else, the staff member who is not immediately available should explain that he or she is not free and that the patient may choose to wait or may choose to return at another time that is agreed. The discomfort that the patient experiences can be subsequently discussed in counselling sessions.

The patient may also have difficulty restraining his or her actions, and, if roused, may act out his or her feelings. For example, a patient who is frustrated may choose to vent his or her frustration on people or property. The clinic should make it clear that such violence will not be tolerated and that the patient will be subject to the penalties imposed on any other member of society who commits a similar act. For example, if a patient damages property, the police should be called and the patient should be charged through the normal legal channels. The magistrate or judge should be advised that, if the patient is convicted, he or she should receive the same penalty (no more and no less) as another person convicted of the same crime who happened not to be an addict.

The matter is complicated because part of the social definition of an illness is that the person is not responsible for the illness (a person with measles does not choose to become infected; a person with schizophrenia does not choose to have auditory hallucinations) and therefore is held to be not fully responsible for actions committed as a direct result of that illness (a person who kills another in response to auditory hallucinations can be deemed under English law as not guilty by reason of insanity or may be deemed to have diminished responsibility). Nevertheless, such a person still receives a disposal from the court (that is, the patient with schizophrenia who is found not guilty by reason of insanity, or found to be guilty but with diminished responsibility, may not be set free from court but rather sent to a secure hospital). On these grounds, if addiction is a disorder, it might be thought that the patient should receive a reduced sentence. But one of the mental functions disordered in addiction is the ability to behave responsibly. Treatment of this disorder of responsibility includes ensuring that the patient experiences the appropriate consequence of his or her action. The clinical staff can then help the patient process what has happened in clinic.

### Projection

But the difficulty taking responsibility leads to subconscious anxiety, which is warded off by the defence mechanism of projection. The blame for an action can be *projected* onto someone else. The drug addict is not an addict because he or she made a choice one day to take a drug but because he or she *was made* addicted by someone else (a doctor who prescribed a pill, a friend who gave it to him or her at a party; society – 'Well, everyone's doing it, aren't they?'). Note the language used here. The basic grammatical structure of most sentences (in English) is in the form:

subject – verb – object

For example Tom hit Fred. The person who is the subject of the sentence (in this example, Tom) carries out the action and is responsible for it. The person who is the object is the innocent bystander. Fred just happened to be in the way and got hit. In conversation with addicts, it is not unusual to find that the addict uses sentences that make the other person (the therapist, the wife, etc.) the subject, with the patient as the object. For example, in the course of discussing what treatment might be appropriate, a patient may say, 'Well, what do you want me to do, doctor?' The unwary doctor will take the cue and prescribe a course of action ('You should go to rehab'). If the patient then goes to rehab, and leaves before completing treatment, he or she can then blame the doctor – 'It's your fault doctor. You told me to go to rehab.' The experienced doctor in the same situation will recognise what is happening and turn the sentence back to the patient. 'What do I want you to do? I don't want you to do anything. The question is what do *you* want to do? The options available to you are ...' In this way, the patient has to make the choice. In such a circumstance, many patients will become annoyed with the doctor for refusing to choose for them, but, after a few encounters of this nature, the patient may eventually come to make a decision themselves.

A variant of this grammar is to put the sentence in the passive form:

'Fred was hit by Tom.'

This can lead the unwary into believing that the speaker is more active than he or she is. For example, a patient may say, 'I was told to see you by my wife.' The patient has made themselves the subject of the sentence, but this use of the passive tense makes it clear that they are *not* choosing to see the therapist.

This example also is an example of projection not only in words but in action. The patient who comes because his wife told him to come will feel that he is not responsible for what happens.

But the use of projection as a defence mechanism is the reason that addicts feel out of control. Their perception (through the spectacles of projection) is that everything that they say or do is not their fault. But, if the fault does not lie within them, the means to remedy the harm that they do is also not available to them. In short, things are not in their control, and they feel out of control. While things are like this, the patient will not be able to recover. Thus the recognition of how the patient cedes control to other people and things and expresses it through language is also a mechanism of assistance in treatment. There is no point making statements like 'You must take control of your life' as the addict does not know how. But showing the patient, gently, by the use of language, how he or she cedes control (and hence abnegates responsibility) allows the patient to learn and take control. And to choose to recover.

While patients are projecting everything outside of themselves, and feel out of control, they feel powerless and worthless. Projection wards off responsibility, but it induces low self-esteem. The patient may then respond to this by reaction-formation (behaving the opposite way to the way he or she feels). They may feel worthless, but behave in a grandiose manner. They may try to increase their own self-esteem by reducing the esteem of others, by sarcasm, hostility, threats and not responding to the requests of others. They may behave as though they are very powerful, with violent outbursts, bullying and even hostage taking. It is clear that, in this situation, attacking the self-esteem of the patient is not likely to result in a desirable outcome.

The patient who projects will feel unable to achieve things by themselves (low self-efficacy). They may responds to this feeling of impotence by fantasising (magical thinking) that they are very capable or that some simple external event will solve everything. In this way, the patient may come to believe that the drug that they use can solve all their problems (notwithstanding the fact that it has harmed them up until now); in treatment, the therapist can be substituted for the drug as the answer to everything.

## Denial

But, if the thought of all the problems gets too much, they can always be denied. Denial involves denying a fact even when manifestly true. As a defence mechanism, it has a place. In its most primitive, denying pain when being chased by a wild animal is crucial, allowing escape to safety. When there is a massive change in circumstances (such as the death of a spouse), denial of that change can allow the mind time to consider and adjust to the new reality. But, when denial persists and prevents action being taken to deal with the harm that is being done, it is no longer healthy. Challenging harshly and directly (as with any defence mechanism) will be followed by stiff resistance, usually in the form of an angry outburst. Where necessary to challenge denial, it is wise to do this gently.

The therapist should express respect for the feelings of the patient and then state that he or she has a different view ('You may say that you only drink socially, but from my point of view you do drink too much'). In this way the therapist is not appearing to try to dominate the patient, who is being treated as an equal. And such equal patients have a right to change their opinion without losing face.

An additional problem with denial is that the patient may make statements that are manifestly untrue. To the outsider, this is lying and evokes feelings of disapproval. In the legal arena, this cannot be tolerated, but in the clinic a more sympathetic approach is appropriate. In this, there is a recognition that not all false statements are malicious. The truth must not be denied by the therapist, but it helps to be aware that there are occasions that patients will make false statements *believing them to be true* because of denial. At other times, patients will intend to deceive. In both these cases, the clinical staff member needs to convey the message that ultimately the patients are deceiving themselves. The staff member will insist on finding the truth and acting on the truth but will not reject the patient every time a falsehood is uttered. If a patient lies, the therapist should indicate that future utterances will not be automatically believed, and that it is up to the patient to rebuild the trust by speaking the truth as far as possible.

But, if a patient is in denial and wishes to avoid reality, two other mechanisms facilitate this. The patient may avoid talk about that reality, even blotting it out in intoxication, or fantasise about things that are most unlikely to happen (magical thinking). The therapist can help by gently reintroducing the truth back into the conversation. If a patient says that he or she will remain abstinent through willpower, it is reasonable to question why he or she should be effective when everyone else who has said the same has failed. A meaningful answer is unlikely, but it may cause the patient to ponder whether the strategy is likely to have a chance of succeeding. At some later stage, the patient can return to discuss strategies of abstinence that are more likely to succeed.

## Summary

Addiction is a disorder with a long period before presentation to the clinic and with a long time required for recovery. Changes can occur only slowly. In the meantime, the patient will go through a process of drug use, then harming themselves and their relationships in accordance with the under-lying dynamics – which they will treat with further drug use.

For the clinician who wishes to help the patient, the vicious cycle needs to be broken, both in the individual encounter and in long-term treatment. People with narcissistic personalities are alexithymic and tend to operate in the area of deed rather than word. Thus, even to the patient who uses intellectualisation as a defence mechanism, treatment of the dynamics requires a focusing by the clinician on the actions of the clinician and the patient. The clinician should recognise the dynamic in the inter-action with the patient on the hospital ward or in the outpatient clinic and not collude with it. The clinician should reinforce boundaries, behave respectfully (but not toadyingly) to the patient with an expectation that the patient will show equal respect, return responsibility to the patient in his or her actions, not in words – save where the addict uses words to enact the dynamic – and assist the patient to learn more mature defence mechanisms to contain his or her own anxiety that will be generated by the clinician behaving in this manner. While the clinicians place great demands on themselves by such behaviour, the likelihood of a successful outcome to the encounter will be greatly enhanced.

## CHAPTER 5

# The psychodynamic assessment of drug addicts

MARTIN WEEGMANN

This chapter is based on the author's assessment experience during the period 1991–1995 with approximately 50 drug addicts at a community drug clinic in London. The majority of these were heroin addicts, both injectors and smokers, though other drugs of abuse, like cocaine or amphetamine and, indeed, multi-drug abuse were common. These assessments were first appointments lasting up to one and a half hours. None of the patients was manifestly intoxicated at presentation, though all were still using illicit substances. By virtue of being psychodynamically guided, these assessments were intended to explore and to formulate a total picture of the role of drug use and addiction in the lives of the individuals concerned and involved some interpretation where possible – either of an exploratory or a containing nature – and among other things a dream was requested. At the same time, there was an emphasis on clarification: What meanings did the drugs have? What was the interpersonal context of using? And, of the referral, how might one begin to situate the person's motivation for help? This contrasted with a more factual or health-focused, active interview carried out subsequently by a doctor. It must be emphasised that such an assessment did not rule out objective or external information about the history of the addiction or social circumstances of the person, but my effort was directed towards building up an impression of the patient's internal world and included consideration of feelings elicited in the assessor; informational aspects were considered important only insofar as they could be tied up to a motivational theme. Such a focus can be overlooked in drug services, which are biased towards a more traditional medical diagnosing, direct questioning or a history-taking attitude in which only conscious material and circumstantial information is sought.

The following is organised under a number of headings, reflecting areas addressed or kept in mind during the actual assessments. We begin, however, with a preliminary discussion of the process of preparation, physical and mental, before the patient arrives.

**Being ready**

Allowing some time to prepare a room, recalling the referral information available and to be physically comfortable all help to promote readiness for the appointment. Some healthcare professionals might feel that it is unduly onerous to pay attention to such time-consuming preparations in the context of a hard-pressed clinic. Much depends, however, on how the agency works and how seriously the assessment process is taken. Is there, for example, sufficient attention given to developing an understanding of the helpful ingredients involved in fostering a therapeutic relationship, even if one only sees the patient once? A chaotic setting can mirror a chaotic patient list and add enormously to the problems of thinking clearly. Too much informality in the assessment (sometimes encouraged by the agency philosophy) can compound the user's casual attitude and difficulty in thinking more seriously about his or her needs. On the other hand, too much formality will alienate and create barriers; so some compromise is needed.

Beyond physical comfort, how does the healthcare professional prepare him- or herself to be mentally ready to see the patient, to be able to take in the experience? Psychodynamic thinking and psychotherapy has had much to say on this topic, usually described in terms of the concept of the 'setting' and on one's initial orientation towards the individual who presents. I will go no further but describe some simple guidelines, which have been written about cogently by Saltzburger-Wittenberg (1970) in her book on psychoanalytic insight and relationships. She identifies four aspects of a basic orientation:

1. **Open-mindedness**. How does one approach the patient without presuppositions? In the author's experience, two problematic assumptions can influence healthcare professionals in the substance-misuse setting: (a) the idea that substance misusers are all the same, making it impossible for the individual's uniqueness to be appreciated and (b) the cynical assumption around expectations of manipulation and deceit. This latter assumption can make it difficult to hear the patient's vulnerability, which may well be heavily defended. At the same time, the healthcare professional needs to have a capacity for healthy scepticism. To be open-minded does not mean to be gullible.
2. **An interest in finding out**. The assessor needs to approach the patient with an even-handed curiosity, both being able to think about the detail and also to think about the overall presentation and referral context. If

preconceived ideas are avoided, the healthcare professional is better able to be receptive to the element of unpredictability inherent in any human encounter.

3. **Listening and waiting**. Closed interviewing does not facilitate good communication, and healthcare professionals should resist a premature wish to formulate an understanding or treatment plan. Miller and Rollnick (1991) refer to the risk of 'premature closure'. This can be difficult when faced with the pressure that the patient may exert for omnipotent understanding and treatment.

4. **Taking feelings and fantasies seriously**. This may seem like an obvious principle of counselling, but in substance misuse the pressure for action can make it difficult to be able to reflect on the feelings involved. Where the individual is engaged in considerable risk taking, the healthcare professional may feel impelled to bring reality to bear; this is indicated in some situations, but, if done prematurely or with moral one-upmanship, further resistance can be encountered.

### The presenting addiction

Addiction could involve substance abuse or substance dependence. In addition to a history of the addiction, a sense of the person's attitude towards it is crucial to ascertain. As with the adage 'Pride goeth before a fall', it is a truism to note that people fight recognition of their addiction for long periods, achieved partly by extensive rationalisation or a creative accounting of the emotional facts. It would seem, from the author's impressions, that at whatever stage of recognition or resistant recognition the person is in, there is normally a double attitude towards the drug, and helping to trace and explore this basic ambivalence is an important first step. In this regard there may be an overlap between psychodynamic approach and the influential approach of 'motivational interviewing' (see Miller and Rollnick 1991 and Weegmann 2002b), which also emphasises the importance of ambivalence, but does so from a more conscious and decisional point of view. Psychotherapy might have more to say on the deeper splits within the individual, which go further than conflicts over whether or not to use substances. A more subtle understanding of motivation has been opened up based on a multifaceted concept of degrees of ambivalence. Freud's observation to the effect that a patient comes to improve his neurosis rather than to cure it could certainly apply to those coming to an addiction service, where the wish for substances without the associated problems is common if not universal (quoted in Spratley 1989). The desire to be the exception and remain in control of drug use is a constant temptation of the addict's thinking.

Some degree of denial towards the addiction and related problems is normally apparent, a denial in particular of the inner significance of problematic experiences or its consequences to others. Perhaps the concept of disavowal is helpful here, insofar as a problem may be recognised at the intellectual level but its emotional significance is separated off. Consider the following example:

> *A patient complained poignantly of what he saw as the stupidity and waste involved in a friend's crack addiction, which had ended his friend's marriage. He seemed, however, remarkably oblivious to the identical dangers in his own situation.*

Sedlack (1989), in his interesting description of disavowal in certain patients during assessment, writes that although 'they were able to communicate to the assessor that their situation was desperate ... They were able to maintain a split between the perception of reality (for example that a psychological disaster had occurred) and the emotional meaning and impact that this has had for them' (p. 99).

## Why now?

This question, concerning what could be described as the 'referral crisis', is linked to the first heading and involves an effort to think with the patient about his or her plight and about the one and only fact about which one can be confident – the fact that they have attended the appointment (though not always on first arrangement or on time). As is well known, the prima facie reasons for attendance are deceptive, for example a patient who talks about a fear of losing their job or relationship if they do not cease drugs may already have been issued such a threat or ultimatum so that a passive situation of having been confronted is turned into an apparently active one with the patient trying to preserve the idea that it is they who are taking the initiative. Eugene O'Neill, in his witty play *The Iceman Cometh* (1947), portrays the various pipe dreams of a group of drinkers, gathered in a Harry Hope's tavern. One character, Jimmy Tomorrow, at one point admits to his distortions. Regarding his job, he says, 'I didn't resign. I was fired for drunkenness', and about his wife he says, 'I pretended it was my wife's adultery that ruined my life. As Hickey guessed, I was a drunkard before that' (p. 195).

Blame and grievance reactions are common, the patient sometimes presenting him- or herself as a victim; perhaps the stance could be likened to that of King Lear in his outcast state, where he regards himself as being 'more sinned against than sinning'.

The question of whose motivation and which part of the person wants to change is important to clarify, a process of thinking by the assessor that should begin even before the initial appointment with the referral circumstance. A patient referred by a partner or the confirmation of the initial appointment by a relative or partner can speak volumes about where, in a family system, the real anxiety is being located. A relative or partner who accompanies the person to their first appointment may, among other things, be making sure that the patient really turns up. The partner may be more worried about the person's use of drugs than the user themselves. I regard a careful inspection of the referral letter, when the patient is professionally referred, as helpful. Take this example:

> A person was referred who had been described by his referring GP as 'draining' to deal with. The patient at assessment appeared to go through the motions of admitting to his drug problems, but his reactions felt shallow and his plans unconvincing. Taking this, together with further information and the benefit of a conversation with the referrer suggested that it was the GP who carried the 'motivation' and that the 'drainage' might have had an economic as well as emotional aspect for his surgery – this being during the transition to the internal market reforms within the National Health Service. It seemed likely that the patient merely wanted his GP off his back.

Often there is a problem in the supply of the illicit drug, and the addict feels cornered. This may be thought of in two ways, which are not mutually exclusive. On the one hand, there is an objective constriction of circumstances – a financial crisis, a threat of violence, legal problems, etc. – which confronts the addict with an untimely obstacle to his or her chosen defence. Unlike a neurotic defence, which is more or less of an internal nature, the addict depends on an artefact and external defence, the drug, and so may be more liable to exposure to such rude awakenings. His or her defences are made up from and are in need of continual reinforcements (further drugs) and in circumstances like these the person may be presenting at a time not of their own choosing. Given this possibility, it is important to gain an impression of when the patient has come to us in order to avoid change rather than to make change. Or, putting this in less stark terms, what aspect of the problem do they identify as being a worry?

On the other hand, this crisis of supply can be regarded as a communication at an emotional level, to the effect that the drugs are becoming an increasingly unreliable container of mental distress. The defensive organisation, pumped and primed by the drugs, is under severe threat, and the person is literally living beyond their psychological means. This could be described not so much as a return of the repressed but a return of the persecutors; indeed, a sense of persecution or a persecutory attitude towards the assessor may well be in evidence in the first meeting. The patient manages to convey his or her drug plight and direct the bad feelings, sometimes into the assessor, and, although change may be wished for, the notion of needing to change is poorly appreciated (see Kernberg et al's 1989 discussion of borderline patients in this regard). As for the shift from one state of mind to another and the breakdown of drug containment, this can be mirrored in how the drug effects are experienced by the user, with a gradual receding of the pleasurable side and an increase in the persecutory side. It is common for heroin users to complain, for instance, that they no longer get a hit or any enjoyment from using.

## The emotional situation

By this term is meant an initial impression of the emotional and cognitive constellation of the patient – their defences, how they think, their schemata, the underlying anxiety and the internal relationship to the addiction. The coverage here, however, will be of necessity a selective one.

Let us start with a patient's dream:

> *An angry female dreamt she was sinking into water that had some rusting metal at the bottom. There was a rotting piece of wood floating by, which she tried to hold onto. Her associations suggested the metal was related to the drugs, needles and the dirtiness of her injecting habit. It was unclear, I speculated, how much she had sunk into the mire and to what extent the dream was a plea for help out of the addiction. But, alternatively has the idea of help already been devalued, like a rotten alternative to the drugs, suggesting the strength of the destructive forces inside her; an important aspect of her presentation turned out to be the wish to be given intravenous opiates from the clinic, which, when refused by the doctor, led to her storming out.*

In a psychodynamic assessment, the emotions conveyed and the emotions aroused in the assessor who is on the receiving end are important to reflect upon, sometimes more so than actual words or details of the story related. Communication is not only by means of words but also by projections in which the person's experience of the assessor, or the clinic which he or she represents, narrows to conform to one restricted perception or another. In the example cited, the patient's overriding attitude was one of blame and grievance – others were to blame for the addiction, starting with grievances towards her parents and so somebody was required to make good; the implied picture of the clinic therefore was narrowed into one of compensating her and subsidising her addiction. We were expected to supply her with drugs decided on her terms, and she saw our refusal to do so as indicating the shallowness of our interest in helping her. The power of the communication was such that the first assessor felt angered by the entitled nature of her demands and the second, who was the doctor who had to say no, felt pushed into guilty feelings and self-justification to manage his refusal of her demands.

Often when the individual presents, perhaps stimulated by growing problems of supply and a decreasing potency of the drug to produce its desired effects, the individual's precarious coping equilibrium is seriously unsettled. Patients in this state may appear overdefended or defenceless and may mobilise difficult feelings in the assessor who sets out to tune into such communications and to empathise.

> *A defended and haughty patient expressed her wariness about the interview, adopting the stance of 'let's get this over and done with, don't detain me'. A difficult atmosphere resulted with enquiry seemingly rejected and the assessor's observations belittled. Later, however, in touching on some precipitating problems, the bravado crumbled and tears filled her eyes. Moments later she wiped these away and started to criticise, as though needing to wipe away any trace of vulnerability and restore her feeling of being in control.*

Aggressive or passive-aggressive defences like these are frequently encountered and could, in part, be viewed as an effort to protect the self from perceived danger. In the chapter on Kohut, for example, aggression or rage is conceptualised as involving a 'narcissistic threat', or an injury to the individual's self. Fonagy et al (1993), writing of certain types of primitive mental functioning, have similarly discussed the role of pathological aggression to fend off threats to the psychological self; they write that, in such personalities, 'Aggression becomes inextricably linked with self expression'(p. 475). It is hypothesised here that the patient at assessment may believe that they have to protect themselves against feelings which have been projected into the outside world so that the recipient (the assessor, the clinic, the consultant, etc.) is viewed as an opposing or a hostile force. This involves the ideas of aggression as a shield and of attack as a principal means of defence, accompanied by an unusually poor ability in such patients to reflect on themselves or their problems. In the straightforward language of NA, 'We tried drugs ... to cope with a hostile world ... The "ultimate problem" was ourselves' (Narcotics Anonymous 1987). Glover (1932), in psychoanalytic language, may have had similar aggressive processes in mind in his classic contribution on drug addiction, in which he describes the addict both as a persecuted and as a persecuting individual.

The metaphor of a retreating army, vividly described by Knight (1953) in relation to the borderline patient, could be applied to this phenomenon of defensive aggression. He describes a military situation in which a few scattered troops or forward detachments protect the bulk of the army and reserves from a state of defeat, retreat or total disarray; their presence on the battlefield gives an illusion of strength. Translating this military metaphor into ego terms, Knight argues that the forward detachments of the army represent the desperate holding operations of a fragile ego, trying to maintain a semblance of control, while the bulk of the ego or ego reserves are in a seriously depleted or tenuous state of existence. Taking this view into the assessment situation, does the patient need to project a fighting front because the underlying situation has become so desperate? After all, as Spratley (1989) reminds us, the patient frequently comes to us in a defeated or rebellious state of mind.

Estela Welldon (1993), writing in the different but related field of assessment for forensic psychotherapy, describes a comparable need to feel in control in forensic patients, for whom their psychic reality may be the opposite and how such individuals fashion a self-survival kit of defences over the years. Within this, she argues, there is a basic attitude of mistrust, desires for revenge and a need to rid themselves of vulnerability.

There may be a category of apparently confident career drug addicts, who may become dealers, just as there are so-called career criminals – and both may share an element of antisocial personality. The following case illustrates how seductive this confidence and control can be:

> *A man spoke eloquently of the damage done by years of drug abuse and his wish to mend his ways. He referred to living on his wits and off the proceeds of crime. Socially, he explained his preference for brief pub-like relationships where he would get to know a lot about someone but would not be known himself. An extended consultation was offered during which he concentrated on various acts of abuse that had been perpetrated by others on him, past and present. There seemed something overassured about his manner, and he dropped out early. In retrospect I wondered whether he had reproduced a brief encounter with me also, from which he then took flight and that his manner illustrated his 'living on his wits' in the transference also.*

With some patients one does not always have the opportunity of seeing powerful emotions but rather a lack of them, and, indeed, it might prove difficult to locate any significant concern whatsoever. It may prove important in interviewing technique to try to intensify the presenting symptoms in order to test the patient's preparedness to think. Needy feelings may seem to be conspicuous by their absence, and such patients are usually described as being in 'precontemplation' in the language of motivational interviewing or 'in denial' in traditional language. I have found the concept of the manic defence helpful here, through which individuals manage to free themselves from real anxiety or depression about themselves – perhaps the drug-taking helps them to dispose of their vulnerability and the related problems are thus removed or felt by others instead. There is little sense of urgency with individuals like this.

> *A patient with a surprisingly casual attitude to the problems she was causing dreamt that she was moving to a large house in which there were several rooms. She linked this jokingly with her circumstances and her disinclination to look after things – she could always move bedrooms once the mess was too great! This patient was, in fact, creating grave concern over her ability to look after herself and her children. Authority and/or people raising their concerns about her were viewed as hostile rather than helpful.*

As an aside, but of interest in the context of patients who evade anxiety, my impression of the dreams reported by drug users is that they frequently suggest an evacuating process in which the dream serves to try to rid the mind of unwanted feelings rather than to make them more available. In terms of asking the patient for their associations to the dream I have been struck by an attitude of indifference or lack of curiosity, which may also link in with the evacuation of unwanted feelings. (See Segal 1986 for a lucid discussion of 'evacuation dreams'; also Flowers and Zwebens's, 1998, excellent discussion of the role of dreams as a valuable treatment resource.) This may link to the use of drugs to evacuate the mind, to kill pain or to produce mental changes without any psychic work – 'changing the way we feel' as people in recovery groups sometimes describe it.

It is not uncommon for patients of this type to present a blandness or a defensive normality in which the person steadfastly refuses to recognise any problems beyond the wish to come off drugs; about the prospects of the latter there is a sanguine attitude, as expressed by two patients thus:

> *All I need from you lot is the kick-start to get off the gear ... you can leave the rest to me.*
> *When I've stopped, there's no way I'm going back to drugs.*

### Current relationships

When asked to describe significant relationships I have been impressed often by the shallowness of the response – descriptions of others sound shadowy, and some patients, for example, merely list a few people or forget to mention children (the latter is more common in men). Significant others appear more likely to be mentioned insofar as they have need-satisfying or problem-bringing qualities: for examples:

> *My mother is the only one to stand by me. She's my tower of strength*
> *I'm getting too much grief off the missus for all this; so I've got to get sorted pretty quick.*

The transference impression of the patient in an assessment can sometimes suggest the person's characteristic way of relating to others. Some patients who become impatient with any process of thinking or questioning, or who adopt a supercilious response to observations, may in their relationships to significant others be derisive, dismissive and tending to blame them for problems, like Jimmy Tomorrow who blamed his wife. This can reflect an egocentrism and an incapacity for deeper relationships so that others become seen as a means to an end:

> 'Look,' said one man after twenty minutes, 'when are we going to get this lot over? I want to know what's going on.' The same man dismissed the suggestion of inviting his partner in, who had confirmed his appointment and came with him and later, when frustrated, walked out saying to his partner, 'Come on; we're going.'

Clearly, much more could be said about the role of relationships and the possible role of co-dependency in partners, not to mention trauma-based family systems (see Chapter 11). This would warrant further, systematic research in view of the suffering that drug addiction is known to cause other family members.

The deeper, internal significance of reported relationships is often difficult to clarify, as the following vignette indicates:

> A patient dreamt a family member was looking over her shoulder while they were in her drug-using area. At first I understood this as an aspect of a benign superego – a helpful figure who was keeping an eye on her. This vaguely linked in with how she presented herself, her charm and apparent earnest attitude. It was only later, when in counselling, that it emerged that the same family member was also a drug-using associate! In retrospect, I wondered whether her presentation had had a seductive and misleading effect on me and that in the dream it was the drug-using part of herself that had to keep an eye on the part of her which was seeking change.

## Past relationships

In assessing drug addicts, I have been impressed by their relative indifference towards talking about the past and wondered whether this was an example of an absence of psychological mindedness. Perhaps it reflects the immediacy of the user's own concerns around his or her own state and suffering. It is often difficult to ascertain any positive sense of the quality of family life and perhaps the past may partly be communicated indirectly through the everyday acting out of drug addiction rather than through conscious recollection. Although the familial past is explored more fully in my later chapter, suffice it here to say that there are frequent reports of the past incidence of a parent(s) with addiction problems, particularly alcoholism, and a variety of other forms of family disorder – violence, neglect or unreliability. These impressions are broadly consistent with the findings of other psychodynamic clinicians, such as Khantzian (1985) and Kaufman (1994). Having said this, one must avoid unhelpful generalisations, and the purpose of asking about past relationships is ultimately to build an impression of what has contributed to the patient being the way he or she is.

### The wish for help

How does the assessor begin to understand the nature of the request for help from the patient? To address this, we need to consider some of the deeper dynamics postulated by some therapists as to the nature of the individual's tie to the drugs.

Writing from a classical viewpoint, Anna Freud (1965a) makes the following point with respect to drug-addicted individuals; she writes, 'The analyst (in our context the "treatment system" of the drug clinic) represents at the same time or in quick alternation either the object of true craving (i.e. the drug itself) or an auxiliary ego called upon to help in the fight against the drug' (1965a, p. 264).

This implies a complex situation, with the drug user in an ambivalent relationship with their drugs – perhaps there is always a struggle of some proportion between the desire to continue the drugs and the desire for freedom from them. Glover (1932), writing yet earlier, has the interesting thought that the 'addiction would represent a peculiar compound of psychic danger and reassurance' – like a good and bad state (p. 319).

By extension, the relationship of the patient to the assessor (what the assessor represents) is ambivalent and perhaps the assessor starts from a position of weakness in not being able to provide immediate relief. At its simplest, why should our goals or abstinence be preferable to their drugs? (See Limentani 1986.)

While this is a poorly understood area, it seems likely that there are gradients of addiction in terms of the underlying emotional situation, which may be quite unrelated to physical dependency as such. With some individuals, for example, one's impression of the addiction is of a complete stranglehold of the drugs and drug thinking over the personality. Here, the drug-taking is completely rationalised, and there is indifference towards the consequences for the self or others. Idealisation of the drugs may be such that a patient may present their addiction not only as a fait accompli but even as a superior state, leading to a challenging situation for the assessor who may feel press-ganged into having to accept rather than being able to question such a perception. In a separate publication (Weegmann 2002a), I describe the aggrandisement of drugs or activities, like gambling, with the building up of a defensive wall around which the individual wards off dissonance or contradiction; the addiction, to use classical language, has become ego syntonic.

At the other end of the spectrum, there are patients who present with less blame and more humility; they seem honest in being able to acknowledge the damage that has been caused and are terrified of adding to it. In other words, there is a fear of being further corrupted by the drugs unless help is sought. Sometimes people present openly with their hands up, acknowledging symbolic defeat in the face of their problems.

To return to Anna Freud's observation, perhaps it is more common to find a kind of intermediate or dual communication, in which the patient successfully manages to convey – including through projective identification – an element of the emotional plight they find themselves in and, at the same time, the paradoxical wish for drug relief from these problems. A patient may urgently want us to know how bad things are but be reluctant or unable to let us help. Help threatens the relationship to the drugs. I would say that at the assessment stage and continuing into, or even throughout treatment, we are faced with a complex three-way negotiation, as shown in Figure 5.1.

At any given moment, and even in the same assessment session, the person may be more or less allied with the clinic or counsellor, and the same applies to the relationship to the drugs.

With respect to the issue of the wish for help, it seems likely that the initial transference is not to the assessor as such but more to what he or she represents: the clinic, the service and the drugs that the service houses. But is the new patient only interested in getting drugs?

Dishonesty in the assessment (of motives, of the amounts and types of drugs used and so on) is not always easy for the professional to fully acknowledge, even when they are aware of its taking place. With a proportion of patients, we know there will be a degree of barter or

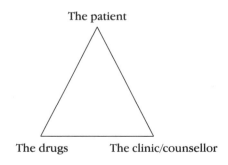

**Figure 5.1:** Three-way negotiation.

coercion in the assessment, and the clinic might be viewed as a corrupt authority which should be worked. Moral manipulation, as with the female patient who was drowning in dirty water, may be a feature of this type of presentation, whereby the healthcare professional is meant to have an uncritical or unreflective sympathy for the patient's point of view. The nature of the setting is, of course, crucial – the patients discussed in this chapter were all seen in a prescribing clinic, which dispenses methadone and other substitute medication. (See Weegmann 1993 for a discussion of some dynamics involved in methadone treatment.)

Ultimately, perhaps our own dilemmas as to what sort of response to offer the drug user (including, but not only concerning, medication) and how we deal with the pressures he or she exerts mirrors an internal dilemma in the user. The demand for relief and fear of the power of the addiction underline the way in which the individual deals with what he or she might regard as being an unequal struggle.

## Conclusion

This chapter offers what is hoped to be a flexible and empathic framework for deepening understanding of how the drug user first presents. Such assessments need to be conceptualised in a bi-directional manner, because, just as we assess the patient, the patient assesses us and will readily pick up on our own state of mind, either of the individual assessor or of the organisation which he or she represents. A psychodynamic orientation highlights the internal world, but does not take away from the importance of considering factual information, the history of the addiction, physical dependence or the familial context. The intrapsychic always needs to be placed in context.

This having been said, the psychodynamic approach nevertheless stresses psychopathology, perhaps in contrast to other approaches that have reacted against such an emphasis or tried to normalise difficulties. Although this is a more practical than theoretical contribution, I would want to distance myself, however, from a reductionist approach prevalent in some psychodynamic writers, with their emphasis on oral dependence, libidinal development or destructive motives only. It is also clear to me that there is a distinction between psychopathology as a background to the development of addiction and psychopathology which results from addiction (see Bean in Bean and Zinberg 1981) and that recovery needs to take account of both. Hopefully, the assessments described here helped our clinic towards a more careful and comprehensive planning of treatment.

# CHAPTER 6

# Psychotherapy with addicted people

## ANNE READ

It is widely believed that it is not possible to work psychotherapeutically with a person who uses drugs; yet, even with someone intoxicated, the presence of someone interested, accessible and non-judgmental may be therapeutic. Consistency and containment gradually replace what has been being sought through drug use and thus allow a space to develop in which an individual can begin to explore themselves, their drug use and its meaning. However, the focus of this chapter is on work with people whose drug use is stable and who wish to reach a point where they feel able to choose to take life on without a buffer, protector, mediator, anaesthetic or any of the other functions a drug fulfils for someone who feels unable to bear what they might call reality without some form of chemical assistance. Joyce McDougall (1989) describes the use of alcohol by one of her patients as 'an attempt to take flight from intolerable affective states' (p. 87). Some patients can only ever tolerate episodes of unformalised therapeutic work within their treatment, but the cases used draw mainly on work with patients seen in formal, weekly, psychodynamic psychotherapy sessions within the context of a drug-treatment programme. Even so some of the work was episodic because the very stress of the therapy at times led to acting out in the form of periods of relapse.

Sedating drugs, heroin and the benzodiazepine tranquillisers, are often described by patients as functioning like 'a cocoon' or 'cotton wool', insulating or numbing the user. They also contain feelings, possibly even preventing psychotic breakdown in some people whose personalities were severely damaged in early life and whose personal resources are unable to manage the resultant disturbance. Stimulants, such as amphetamine and cocaine, increase sociability and lift the user above feelings making, as it were, a layer of ice between consciousness and pain and thus function as antidepressants. Khantzian's 'self-medication hypothesis' sees the user finding their drug of choice accidentally through experimentation but recognising it because of its effect of bringing the user into a more desirable state by containing or correcting distressing feelings (Khantzian 1977). For many addicted people, their drug permeates their lives, offering a relationship in its own right and providing occupation in the process of obtaining it and the money to buy it by fair means or foul and thus defining their place in society. Drugs become the devil they know, with effects that are predictable, rapid in onset, under their control and independent of others. They are akin to the Winnicott's 'transitional object' (Winnicott 1951) but link the user to themselves, ultimately, and not to another. They give them an identity as an addict, and this identity protects them from both past and future.

Few drug users seek psychotherapy or can afford private treatment while few private therapists will (or should) feel comfortable allowing a person heavily involved in the drug scene into their relatively unsecured consulting rooms. Most drug users present to drug-treatment services asking for a substitute prescription. The question of abstinence often arouses enormous ambivalence after years of dependency, and services often collude by taking the drug as the problem. The quality of the individual's story and experience of life may never be explored, and this avoidance echoes society's ambivalence towards the addicted person as well as that person's ambivalence towards themselves.

People do not become addicted without reason. Drug services now recognise that the majority of their clientele have suffered emotional, physical or sexual abuse in childhood. They may have lived with violent or addicted adults or been taken away from them into a care that is uncaring and where they may have been abused, or they may have failed educationally or in the establishment of themselves as self-determining adults. It is acknowledged that they have a higher incidence of psychological and psychiatric problems than the general population (Khantzian and Treece 1985). Such people lack the self-esteem and ability to trust others, qualities which are necessary in order to establish a place in the world and make adult relationships. Also drug use may be a survival mechanism, however maladaptive. In my view, many of my patients would probably have killed themselves through either suicide or lack of self-care had they not become dependent.

Psychotherapy with drug users therefore raises the same issues as work with any seriously damaged and maladaptively defended patient. Ambivalence, distrust and dependency can be extreme and testing, challenging and recurrent. The work may be lengthy, and the therapist must tolerate periods of absence and chaos while maintaining consistency.

In addition, the drug, as relationship and as defence, is a concrete presence in the patient's bloodstream and state of consciousness that they have come to need in order to function. This must be acknowledged in the work and recognised in the acting out, since drugs then constitute a practical and possibly life-threatening danger that forces the therapist to tread a fine line when assessing, reflecting and acting on the risks to the patient or to others. It is difficult to contain one's concern, not be non-judgmental to the point of being unrealistic and yet convey to the patient an understanding of their need for their drug. People use drugs to avoid painful feelings, thoughts and memories, producing a chemical dissoci-ation, and the therapist can experience intense feelings while the patient is cut off, calm and unaware of what is happening in the unconscious. Drug use can also reduce impulse control and allow the explosive release of otherwise suppressed emotion. Patient and therapist must recognise that both situations are possible in order to be prepared to work with and contain them safely.

**The drug as container**

Telling one's story for the first time can bring relief, because someone has cared to listen and wanted to know, but there may be a fear that the hearer will not take the knowledge seriously, will disbelieve, react punitively or judgmentally or use it against one. Feelings of exposure and vulnerability may be terrifying, and the therapist's interest may even be seen as intrusive. This may lead to an episode of exacerbated drug use, which can drop both user and therapist into failure and hopelessness. The need is for understanding, containment and tolerance without condoning the self-harm inherent in the chaos while the therapist is tested for their ability to recognise and help bear the pain and to carry the hope that a human relationship can replace drug use.

Heidi's tranquilliser use had reached the point where she was taking pills in handfuls, was so disinhibited that she was often violent, had become a prostitute in order to buy supplies and had taken several, semi-intentional, severe overdoses. She had previously seen a child psychiatrist, and her notes gave me the opportunity to ask why, at the age of seven, she had thrown faeces out of her bedroom window. Her answer was that she was locked in. Her story was that she had been adopted by a professional couple and used regularly by her father for sex. Her mother, aware of this, blamed Heidi, who acted out her distress with tantrums at home and disruptive behaviour at school, which led to the child-psychiatry referral. When I asked why she had not said that she was locked in, she said that they had not asked. No one ever had, and her mother's treatment had led her to believe that telling would make no difference. She only expected to be seen as bad, untruthful and unlovable. She could not bear or understand her feelings or control them, having never been shown how to do so, as Krystal shows in his description of alexythymia in drug users (Krystal 1982). In her teens she discovered that tranquillisers numbed her rage and despair and, by the time that we met, could not imagine living without them.

Containment first meant setting boundaries to her drug use with a prescription so that the drugs and the drugs service began to share her dependency. Further disclosures followed, and for the first couple of years each episode of telling, understanding and being understood was succeeded by a retreat into chaos where Heidi regained a sense of control of her life by buying drugs illicitly again. Prescribing was stopped until it became safe; appointments with the therapist were not. The therapeutic message was 'I am here, do not like what you are doing to yourself, but understand and am not rejecting you.' With time, this could be put into words, and the words heard until Heidi came to trust the therapist, value herself and stop the prescription. She is now at university where she is preparing to use her experience, thereby validating it, since living without drugs means that she must contain what she knows in some other way, which, for her, is helping others and developing her own understanding.

### The drug as substitute

I once asked a heroin user what heroin meant to him; he put a melodramatic hand on his heart, tipped his head back and howled 'mother'. He knew that he was acting and that he was too afraid of what he was saying and its implications to be able to say it without self-mockery. Another man described heroin as 'the White Lady: completely beautiful, utterly warm and impossibly perfect' in a dreamy voice with eyes closed; with eyes open, there was no eye contact. People who have not been wanted or felt unloved have a terrible sense of absence, which they may describe as yearning, as hunger or as a black hole. It demands filling through relatedness, yet they do not know how, and filling the emptiness with drug use feels safer and easier. Relationships with a therapist will be problematic, evoking past despair, abuse, failure, never-met dependency needs, grief and inevitable ambivalence.

Isabel was a middle-class child whose mother could not love her and projected her own sense of failure into her daughter in the form of dislike. Perfection was expected, and so she always felt that she failed. An affectionate child, she was rebuffed whenever she tried to give or receive cuddles or affection. Her father, largely absent with work or other women, had a cold, functional relationship with her mother. His interest in Isabel was only in her scholastic achievements; she said, 'He only wanted me to boast about to his friends.' In her teens, her mother took her to Weightwatchers calling her daughter's developing body 'fat'. She began starving, trying to look perfect and thus be loveable. Purging and vomiting made her feel 'light and clean inside'. The GP, where her mother took her next, treated her with Valium; this dulled her feelings of inadequacy and self-dislike and made her awkwardness seem to matter less. She began a double life, gaining O levels and A levels while furiously rebelling against her mother in order to go to night clubs where she drank heavily and used drugs. Instead of going to university, she enjoyed disappointing her father by moving in with an older boyfriend who made her feel grown up and important but was a heroin dealer who treated her with contempt until she tried the drug. She said, 'It made me feel warm all the way through inside for the first time in my life.' She became addicted rapidly while her partner took perverse pleasure in injecting her.

By her early twenties, her partner was in prison, and she had taken over his drug-dealing business. She was not sure why she had come for help, but drugs were losing their effect, and she had begun bingeing and vomiting again. Very thin, with huge dark eyes, abscesses on her arms and a rigid politeness, she said that she thought that she was going mad and was considering suicide but, having not yet come to a final decision, she was prepared meanwhile to accept a substitute prescription. This was easily arranged but only on condition that she gave up dealing, leaving her much empty time and nothing to fill it with. As she said, that felt like the story of her life. I suggested she might want to talk about that story with a view to making some sense of it. The therapy lasted almost three years.

At first Isabel was quite frozen, sitting watchfully opposite me and scything through my questions and reflections with icy contempt. She was, of course, always neat, punctual and polite, and I felt inadequate in my total inability to get through to her. I had nothing to offer; she was complete in her comforting drug use, and I could not touch her despair, though occasionally, briefly, I saw the loneliness and despondency in her eyes. One day she came on foot and arrived cold and wet; I offered a cup of coffee and suggested she move her chair towards the radiator. She refused irritably, and I wondered out loud if I might be feeling a little as she used to as a child with her mother. She looked at me with amazement and said that she did not suppose I was feeling anything at all; I asked if she had ever felt that she could affect her mother in any way. She burst into tears and sobbed for the rest of that session; the next were filled with story after story of childhood loneliness and her belief that it would never end. Between accounts, she was stiff and cool, apologising for wasting my time complaining when she should be sorting her life out, but now she could hear that this was precisely what she was doing in allowing herself to feel feelings that had been frozen first by her mother and then by her drug and alcohol use. She had never believed that she could be accepted by anybody good and so had made do with people whom she saw as being as unlikeable as herself.

I became, in transference, the perfect mother whose approval she must ensure with flowers and little cakes and sweets that she made herself. She reduced her prescription and would not hear my concern that she was doing so faster than she could manage while still very vulnerable. When she visited her mother for her birthday I was not surprised that a disastrous attempt to gain her mother's love, with a cake and beautifully wrapped presents that were disparaged by her mother as 'home-made', led to a serious overdose. That she did not die allowed us to work with the part of her that wished she had. She felt that the absence at the centre of herself, which she now knew to be her mother's, was taking her over, and spent long periods in sessions curled up in a foetal position saying nothing. I had to let her know that I could wait for her without making her feel either abandoned or chivvied and that I would not blame her for dying if that were her choice. I also had to contain my own anxiety while still letting her know that I cared and was concerned for her. Her own birthday came and with it another overdose, after which she reluctantly accepted a stay in hospital. Here, in the art-therapy room, though she would not join the group or accept individual sessions (thus keeping me as the only person who was allowed to know how she felt and, as she later admitted, ensuring my continued anxiety on her behalf), she began to experiment with paint and clay. She made an array of models of herself at different ages and in different moods and was delighted to be allowed to take them home when she was discharged, arranging them carefully on her mantelpiece where the kitten could not harm them. 'What kitten?' I asked, and she said that it had 'adopted' her 'so now I can't kill myself, because then who would look after it?' I was now sharing with a kitten the responsibility of keeping Isabel alive while she began to integrate all the frozen hurt now embodied in her little clay creations.

Once again she began to reduce her prescription, this time slowly and demanding breaks in the reduction to test my trust in her to begin to know for herself what she needed. She made new friends in a craft workshop where she began to make clay figures for sale. She even put on a little weight and bought new clothes. She was asked to help in a playgroup and discovered a talent with children. All these new discoveries and successes both overjoyed and terrified her, and she had outbursts in which she smashed her possessions and tore her pretty new clothes; it was very hard for her to accept that this was her rightful rage with her parents which she was turning on herself because she felt powerless to touch them. The small children in the playgroup were showing her what childhood should be like, and it hurt. Suddenly, I could do nothing right; my every word, question, thought and interpretation was wrong. She would miss sessions, saying that therapy was no good and that she was too busy to come or rage at me for being unable to change an appointment at short notice. She did not stop working in the playgroup, however, and continued to make and sell her little figures. I remembered that her mother's birthday was approaching again, and she exploded at me for not having realised that earlier – 'How could you be so stupid?' – and then cried heartbrokenly. We could now agree that I had had to accept the anger from her that her mother never would and that we had both lived through the experience.

The rest of her therapy was reasonably smooth; Isabel stopped her prescription and, when some of her new student friends invited her to move in with them, she did so and obtained a place on a course to train to work with children. She had a difficult time when her old partner was released from prison but allowed her friends to look after her and even to remind her to eat.

### The drug as identity

People who have been sexually abused in childhood, particularly if there has been violence or sadism or the abuse began early, often have an extremely fragmented or distorted sense of self or none at all. Their internal world can be split between abused and abuser, and they may either identify with or be caught up in the cycle of abuse and self-abuse without any sense of identity. Someone who repeatedly abuses children is addicted to this process, and the children are the object of the addiction – in effect, the abuser's drug. They may even be drugged to make them tractable, and their whole family may be involved, rendering the child unable to find help even if they are not too intimidated. For such children, the whole world is abuse, and, if drugged, the periods of sedation may be their only comfort.

Cora was one such child. Her parents came from families in an organised paedophile ring operating in each other's houses and an old church. Cora was taken there once a week and both experienced and witnessed extreme sexual sadism and torture. Her father raped her regularly at night, and her mother used her by day as a skivvy and beat her. Meanwhile, her father had a respectable job, the children were well-dressed and went to school, and the family went to church on Sunday. School, with its normal rules and limits, was the one sane place in Cora's life; there she could protest, and her behaviour frequently got her excluded but no one was able to persuade her to say what was wrong, because she was too afraid of punishment from the ring, too involved with the family's perverse standard of loyalty and totally unable to imagine herself living normally.

Nonetheless, perhaps because of her own strong character and her need to defend others if she could not defend herself, perhaps because she once overheard her grandmother saying that her father 'treated the maid cruel', Cora knew that what she saw and went through was wrong. She held onto that knowledge and blamed herself for being unable to act on it. At fourteen she became pregnant and miscarried the baby when her father kicked her, at sixteen she went to police college as a cadet in order to escape, broke down, was discharged and took various jobs, including prostitution where she met drug users. Amphetamine suited her, and she 'became the life and soul of the party'. For the first time she could contain and cut off her pain, memories and flashbacks, make friends and enjoy herself. For seven years she forgot until, half-intentionally, she became pregnant again. She gave up drugs for the sake of her baby and returned to the verge of breakdown. For her child's sake, since having no sense of self she could not seek it for her own, she came for help.

Therapy was in two parts, separated by a major breakdown which hospitalised her for a year when her daughter was seven, the age at which Cora's own conscious memories began. For a long time, she had no sense of herself as a person, but only a story to tell. This was told haltingly with the therapist being challenged at each tiny step to believe and disbelieve simultaneously. Belief would make it real and thus unbearable. Disbelief would thrust Cora back into lonely non-existence. Neither was bearable for long, and she could tolerate no show of emotion in herself or her therapist; she punctuated her therapy with episodes of clinically effective, illicit amphetamine use. Any offer of a prescription was rejected; the therapist had to accept that this self-abuse was the only survival stratagem that Cora could accept, her only way of retaining control and avoiding breakdown into the madness that terrified her. Gradually, she came to believe herself and, as a sense of self began to form, increasingly blamed and hated herself. She was the abuse. She deserved the abuse. She was abusive. She had known that it was wrong and done nothing. These ideas were held with a fixity fuelled by her terror at having no sense of control in the present, having had none in the past. She felt herself to be harmful to both her daughter and her therapist and took an overdose in order to protect them.

Even though the therapist, whom I supervised, was able to understand the underlying mechanisms, Cora's beliefs were held with too much psychotic intensity to be worked with, and we admitted her to hospital. We knew that, if she abandoned her belief in her own dangerousness prematurely, she would have nothing with which to defend her underlying sense of total exposure, betrayal, brokenness and horror. She would once again be nothing. Unless identified with the abuse and the abuser, she had no sense of power or identity. Hospital was a retreat where she regressed and made brief, painful contact with feelings of helplessness and neediness interspersed with suicidal despair or cold hostility. She came to understand that these feelings were the reality of her childhood and began to grieve.

Leaving hospital, she gave up drug use and went to study law, taking a break from therapy to 'just live'. She returned because, although successful, she felt 'like an actress and not like a real woman'. Her therapist had moved, and I took up the work. Cora felt that she had to invent everything she did and, although everyone else was convinced, she felt quite unreal. I wondered whether her reality was rooted in the paedophile ring, leaving her no sense of goodness – and therefore her own goodness – as having any truth to it. 'I did not need to hear that,' she said, coldly hating being seen in any way as good. Once again, she was identified with her abuse but this time could stay sane and work with it without drugs.

One day her computer broke down and the engineer treated her 'like a stupid little woman'. She knew that it was not her fault and was able to prove it. When the engineer left, she cried and cried for the child who had believed that everything was all her fault and was not hard at all, but soft, sensitive, caring and trapped. I was allowed to validate that and to hear about, but not witness, her tears. She forgave the child she had been but still not the adolescent who had allowed her father to kill her pregnancy while she had been unable to leave the ring where she repeatedly witnessed and was forced to participate in the abuse of other children. It took many more storms, but no more breakdowns, before she could see that she had been the object of abuse – the drug – and not an abuser and that without a sense of self, other than as abusive and with no expectation of being believed if she spoke of the ring, she could not escape until she found a container – the police force – powerful enough to lend her a sense of control. She then began to integrate a sense of identity, survival and value and to know that she could look after herself and her daughter safely. She had shown someone her world, and they had been able to give her a true reflection of herself in it.

## The dance with death

For a person deeply involved with drug use, death need never be far away. This can be a comfort since, just as drugs deaden feeling and memory, they can be an exit if life becomes completely unbearable or pointless. When the inner world cannot love life, death may be loved in its place. Others have an inner world so deadened by neglect or abuse that they only feel alive in extremes; these gamble with drug use and other forms of self-harm, deriving stimulus from danger and becoming addicted as much to that as to the drugs. They may also seek the disinhibiting effect that can produce an extreme state of false courage, overcoming the fear of life in an illusion of power, control and confidence. The process of using a drug can be a ritual in which the preparation for taking it is as important as its effect. 'The unconscious model underlying drug use', says Zoja (1989), 'has a religious tint ... That of the Lost Paradise' (p. 66). People speak of a heightened awareness, of feeling outside time and in another world where they have everything that they need and they do not need anybody. They feel complete and reach a state that some compare with orgasm and others call mystical; they are with the White Lady, who may be Death or *la petite mort*. Yet this ritual of transition or transformation can never be complete and so they always have to return, always try again.

Drug use can also be an unconscious way of keeping death at bay. Jane requested psychotherapy about five years after I had treated her alcoholism because she had begun drinking again. During her previous treatment, she had spoken of a lonely childhood with an angry, disappointed mother, divorced from an intellectual, professional man who sent her to boarding school and whom she only saw in the holidays. Later she became addicted to heroin but had given it up, married, set up a business and had a daughter. She could not understand why, with everything she had wished for now present in her life, she had become an alcoholic. I suggested psychotherapy to explore this, but she was terrified at the thought and fled into health.

She returned because she was using drink consciously to deaden what threatened to be overwhelming feelings of despair, even though her life was going well. Jane felt that she had to understand herself and brought a palpable anxiety into the room that I could not help but share; we agreed that it had a desperate urgency and felt very deep.

She started to tell me her dreams. She was being breast-fed, and it felt good. We thought that we had made a safe place from which to begin. Then she was pushing a boat out to sea and alone in it with her father in the dark but could not explain the accompanying sense of dread. Her father had been dead for many years, and I grew concerned; when she said that she was experiencing episodes of breathlessness, I urged her to see her GP. I was reminded of a patient of whom Joyce McDougall (1986) writes and for whom cigarettes were 'a life-threatening addiction [with] an unconscious fantasy of joining his dead father ... to protect himself from his stifling mother' (p. 89). I suggested a break in therapy to allow her to rest, but she could not bear the idea, becoming even more anxious and so we continued. Then her brother told her of being sexually abused in childhood by their father and his second wife, and Jane had a dream in which the wife said to the father, 'Of course, Jane is totally destroyed.' She looked at me for a long time and then said slowly, as if describing a picture, 'All those cameras.'

The dread and horror which filled me must have been hers as well as mine. I was shocked but not surprised when her partner telephoned to say that Jane had suffered a massive pulmonary embolus. She asked me to visit her, and we agreed that, although we had only had ten sessions, her urgency now seemed to make sense. Or had we done something that we should not have and unleashed an illness that was being held in check by chemical defences? Her partner telephoned a few days later to say that Jane had gradually weakened and died; he also said that she had been more at peace than he had ever known her and that 'it was a good death'. Maybe therapy had had some part in that or perhaps it was death itself that had brought peace. And perhaps Jane's sense of urgency and the rapidity with which she went to the heart of things were due to an unconscious awareness of how little time she had.

Jim had also been to boarding school, one for children whose families could not contain them. He described himself as the black sheep of his family and could not excuse them enough for their inability to set safe limits to his behaviour. By his teens he was chaotically using alcohol, amphetamines and whatever pills he was offered by his older friends, and his criminal behaviour was increasingly challenging. He was put into care and by his late teens had nearly died several times. He presented two sides: one was bright and entertaining, and it was difficult not to be seduced by it and spend whole sessions in puns, mimicry and hilarious stories. The other was terrified of the night, and Jim did everything he could to avoid the sleep in which he would invariably dream to be awoken sweating and yet still in the dream. He had a recurring nightmare in which two huge men forced their way into his bedroom in order to rape and kill him.

Psychotherapy meant episodes of work interspersed with chaos, but each group of sessions produced small gains of trust and understanding. We agreed that we would work with the pattern but that, if he were intoxicated, he would telephone to arrange another time. He was able to honour this agreement and to see that it honoured him. He spoke of his schooldays where boarding school had felt safer than life with alcoholic parents. Gradually, he revealed that the teachers had their pick of the children for sex and the children competed with each other to be chosen. He was amazed when I stated that that was abuse and that it made me very angry on his behalf; he had never realised that it was wrong. I wondered why he had been unable to know and probably asked too soon, because he withdrew. I wrote to him, but received no reply.

When he did make contact, he told me defiantly that he had been 'back on the game' and using drugs. He waited for my response, for once without flirting with me. When I said that I was angry not with him but with the self-abuse being acted out in him, he admitted to being frightened by the degree of risk he had taken. He then produced an old school photograph, saying, 'There I am, only fourteen. I thought I was so mature, but I'm only a child, aren't I?' Indeed he was – a very beautiful, vulnerable child, and I told him so. He became very quiet and then cried softly for a long while, saying, 'I never realised before that it was wrong.'

He dreamed again; there was only one rapist in the room, and Jim could see past him to the door but did not know whether he would be able to reach it. He attended the sessions less regularly but without the same extremes of chaos and then told me he had fallen in love with an older man, alcoholic but not abusive, who understood him. He did not want more therapy; he wanted to just live and enjoy life. I have not heard from him since and so do not know who the second rapist might be or whether he or the alcoholic partner is linked with Jim's early life, nor do I know if Jim will be able to keep away from life-threatening drug use without that knowledge. I have to wait and see if he will need or be able to come back.

**Transference and countertransference**

Patients often expect therapy to work like a drug, producing rapid gratification, a predictable response and good feelings; they can easily feel let down or betrayed when it does not. The projection may extend to the therapist who is seen either as the dealer (particularly if they work in a prescribing service) or actually as the drug, making them feel withholding, unreal, treacherous or all three. An addicted person inhabits an all-or-nothing world; they feel good or they feel bad. If the badness is internalised, they feel themselves to be all bad and project goodness, expecting judgement, condemnation and deprivation. If they reject past adverse experience, the world (in the person of the therapist) is hurtful. The swing between these two primitive positions can be bewilderingly rapid when the effect of the therapy in the role of the drug is not instantly forthcoming. The therapist will swing between feeling the most important object in their patient's world and feeling useless, valueless and written off. Each position feels, and is, unreal; the drug or the need for it is mediating the relationship. It is the drug that is expected to have the effect, and it lacks the subtlety and individuality of human relationship.

There is no space for negotiation, question or compromise. The drug is the token of exchange and dictates value. In effect, there are three in the work, and the therapist is seen as in control, able to give or withhold reward: a dealer. The patient attempts to obtain the reward: the good feeling. One patient, stable on his prescription, reasoned with me that 'I have been good; so I deserve an increase'. Another did not believe me capable of even such a 'straight' deal and offered to deposit a large sum of 'inherited' money in my bank account for my children. He was incredulous when I said that I was not a laundry; I was supposed to feel complimented!

A therapist faced with such non-negotiable absolutes, expectations and projections easily feels unskilled; one may be a persecutor who does not understand, a victim in the face of the patient's censure or not even a person but a substance. Finding a place from which to work is hard, as is maintaining consistency. It is tempting to give and give in order to remain a good object or to become angry with repeated rejection and disempowerment. When one feels treated as a drug or drug dealer, it is easy to miss the desperation of someone who cannot deal with people directly and feels exposed without their drug and their dealing.

Exposure and shame are crucial. Many drug users have been given, and have taken, the role of black sheep. Some are addicted to abuse, having known little else in the way of stimulus or notice. Shame may be intrinsic and the devil they know; to contemplate giving it up is terrifying, and having it exposed feels irreparable. It is as though there is no good option, and they can become horribly stuck while the therapist desperately tolerates ambiguity and waits for despair to find a voice. When it does, it is utterly demanding and does not know how to wait. A young woman would drop into the waiting room and sit there for hours. She was quiet and the receptionist tolerant; each time I came out of my office to fetch a patient, I would smile and speak briefly. In our sessions she raged at me for not giving her unbooked time, and I felt guilty and mean. Gradually, she realised that I was there, did keep my word and did genuinely acknowledge her existence even when it was not her session. I was not, and was not like, her punitive mother and exploitative father and would not let her behave like them towards me; she could choose to share the boundaries I offered as a safe place within which to work.

Drug use may be an escape from the need for change when change feels impossible. An unconscious need for transition can fix on the actual experience of intoxication as a ritual, a rite of passage or even a death and rebirth process that is never completed, since the patient returns unchanged. Drug use becomes more and more extreme, and the pseudo-ritual is invested with reality while the risk itself is needed in order to feel alive, a brink from which the user may not return easily, if at all. The therapist has to preserve a place for reality until the process can be interpreted and understood. It is frustrating and demoralising to be a mere human being offering an experience of relationship and understanding that seems so much less glamorous and exciting than that offered by drug use, but it is real. The rite of passage through the drug is illusory and does not alter its user's place in the world. It is exclusive, and the therapist will know that it is being relinquished when they no longer feel shut out. The task is then to support the patient in their struggle to be ordinary and to make a real life.

It is as necessary to know why one chooses to work with addiction as it is to know why one chose to become a therapist. One must understand one's own attraction to risk-taking and dependency needs, since otherwise one is in danger of seduction by larger-than-life illusions and all-or-nothing extremes. This may reflect society's fascination with addiction which is both vilified and glamorised in a way that much deviant behaviour is not; drug users are outside of both the law and society and many welcome this familiar placing. Identity and belonging are projected onto the drug scene, and society is expected to reject. Society reciprocates with stigma. Perhaps the addict mirrors society's fascination with consumption. Luigi Zoja (1989) writes of an attitude of the drug addict 'which does not belong to him alone but to all of society ... a close analogy between addiction and consumeristic behaviour' (p. 93); this is a view of itself that society strives to avoid. A therapist working with addicted people has to be able to avoid identifying with either attitude and yet be able to understand both in order to help their patients to make a real transition.

If the therapist can do this, and can tolerate the necessity of breaks in the work should the patient's drug use become chaotic or life-threatening, the patient is enabled to work through and out of their addiction and make a place in society. In addition, a psychodynamic understanding in a drug service informs the counselling that must be available to all its patients and, in a less formal way, enhances the treatment of many more.

# CHAPTER 7

# Group therapy for addiction

JAMES MOSSE AND MARY ANN LYSAGHT

## Introduction

This chapter draws on over five years' experience of our providing group therapy for people with problems of drug or alcohol abuse. In the group we did not distinguish between alcohol and other drugs (nor do we in this paper), and many members had problems with both. The groups were run on psychoanalytically informed lines at an inner-city clinic and met once weekly for one and a half hours. We aimed to provide longer-term treatment to patients returning to independent living after detoxification or a period in a rehabilitation programme. They were slow, open groups (that is, open-ended rather than fixed-term and with the expectation that old members would leave and new members join over the life of the group). When new members joined, they were told that there were only four rules: they must attend every week, they must give the group four weeks' notice of their intention to leave, members must not meet or socialise outside the group and there was to be no physical violence in the group. This last rule was always presented as being not just a prohibition but also an assurance that others would not be permitted to be violent towards them.

We did not have a rule requiring members to be abstinent, though we did have a firm stance that they must be motivated to give up using drugs if the group was to be of any help to them. Thus we did not accept new members who were currently addicted or heavily drug-dependent. Existing members who relapsed or binged, however, were not asked to leave the group; so there were frequently both using and non-using members simultaneously. Our not insisting on abstinence differs from the stance taken by many other healthcare professionals, and with hindsight we feel that it had both advantages and disadvantages. We discuss below the thinking that lay behind this and other choices that we made and, importantly, our retrospective conclusions about the project and the lessons we have learned from it.

## Understanding the problem

We believe that in addiction drug use is not the fundamental problem requiring treatment – many addicts have had significant drug-free periods, but have then relapsed. Our view is that addiction is an attempted solution to an unbearable internal state, a view that differs from a predominantly biological understanding, which would give more weight to an innate genetic or biochemical predisposition. Psychodynamically, the causes of addiction are complex and multiform, and the severity of the underlying psychopathology can vary considerably, but we think that it is important to try to understand the nature of the developmental disturbance that the addictive substance is supposed to assuage.

Psychoanalytic literature provides a wealth of understanding of both the psychopathology of addiction and the meaning of drug use. The type of person we are discussing is variously identified as manic-depressive, narcissistic, pathologically dependent and having a weak ego. Addicts are found to have suffered serious deprivation early in life, often with parents who were unable to put the children's needs first, even projecting their own disturbance and extreme dependence onto the child. Consequently, as the personality of the addict develops it is both weak and beset by primitive emotional states of intense need and impulsive aggression. This is because the mental equipment that might allow the toleration of psychic pain has never developed in the absence of a containing parental figure. The loss, mourning and bearing of depressive affect that normally supports a coming-to-terms with the reality of separateness and individuation instead carries for the addict the threat of overwhelming depression or breakdown, felt as a return to childhood trauma. This sets the stage for turning to drugs in an attempt to alleviate or take control of painful states of mind arising from an internal deficit that is experienced as unbearable. It is notable that almost all of our group members had appalling early lives, frequently with traumatic loss and often with horrific abuse. It is likely that such distorted and persecuting early experiences greatly increased the pressure to turn to primitive defences, such as splitting, and militated against successful subsequent reintegration of these splits.

Herbert Rosenfeld (1965) makes an important contribution to the understanding of addiction when he notes the way in which drugs support and reinforce manic-depressive defences in a personality that would otherwise be too weak to uphold them. He believes that addicts regress not to the realistic dependence of the infant at the breast but to the narcissistic pseudo-independence of thumb sucking (to which he equated drug use) and its support of hallucinatory wish fulfilment. Thus, the primary external figure of dependence (who may in reality have been unbearably undependable) is replaced by a sense of total self-sufficiency. In the infant this is achieved at the cost of an associated denigration of the feeding breast and, as the years progress, of all later relationships of potentially benign dependence. This thesis helps us to understand a clinical presentation that often includes a pull towards narcissistic withdrawal or manic triumph over salient figures, such as therapists, simultaneously with an intense hunger for the relationship. Later in the chapter we will illustrate this ambivalent picture as it was presented in relation to the groups we provided.

## Case studies

Our first vignette illustrates how addicts seek to defend themselves against the awful anxieties and pressures of their poor internal state by having recourse to manic mechanisms that, with their weak ego, can only be sustained by drug use.

### Linda

Linda was a group member who had a twenty-five-year history of varied drug abuse, primarily as a cocaine and then a heroin addict. She had remained clean for many years but had recently relapsed as a consequence of difficulties at work. She went on holiday to stay with an ex-addict friend who had gone to live abroad to try to get away from drugs. This was a location supposedly free of hard drugs, and Linda was convinced beforehand that, by going to stay there, she too would be able to give up heroin. On her return she told us that in fact crack cocaine had been freely available, and her friend had been using heavily. Linda had used compulsively throughout her vacation and had then bought more crack cocaine to smoke on the plane home. She had some left over, which she decided to risk taking through customs and finish up on the train into London. Another member of the group, Jack, laughed collusively at this recklessness, although the picture Linda presented was awful and full of unacknowledged despair. He said that he had been drinking all week and thought that he was liable to be arrested for doing something mad.

We can see in this vignette the way in which Linda first pursues an idealised magic solution (that by changing location she can change her habit), but, when this fails her, she is overwhelmed by despair from which she takes flight into drug use. The effects of the drug then directly reinforce this manic escape mechanism. Both she and Jack had very little inner control and then placed themselves in situations that invited external authority (customs or police) to intervene and punish them harshly.

The poor capacity to parent themselves and the inability to bear mental pain has left such patients prone to the use of manic defences, such as idealisation and identification with an ideal object. These mechanisms are used to control both paranoid and depressive anxieties, with the drug felt to be an ideal substance that can be concretely incorporated. In addition, the resulting high reinforces omnipotent denial of guilt and anxiety. Thus the drug seemingly annihilates internal frustration and persecution, though one can simultaneously see the risks taken as a wish to elicit punishment from an external authority for both the internal and the external out-of-control state. This may reflect a healthy impetus to put a stop to omnipotent destructiveness alongside a more masochistic wish to invite retribution against the self.

*Tony*

Tony was a group member who was renowned for being workshy and had tested his employer's tolerance to the limit with repeated episodes of sick-leave, usually associated with hangovers. One day he described how a colleague at work had not been doing the work that the manager was giving him. Tony said that he was not going to cover up for the skiver any longer (which he had been), nor was he going to defend him to management, even though Tony was the union representative. It would seem here that, although still projected, there is recognition of the skiver in himself, which he seems to be prepared to tackle by acknowledging the reality of the situation. At this point, after his passive-aggressive tendency to lie to and trick his employers had been repeatedly addressed in the group, he seems to have the beginnings of an internalisation of a benign authority, non-persecuting but honest, which he can turn to in himself.

### Inability to internalise

The addicts' basic problem, which dominates their psychic reality, is the inability to internalise adequately an experience of good relationships with others in a way that allows these to be turned into inner resources. There are several possible contributors to this state. The capacity to inter-nalise may be weakened because the externalising projective tendency predominates. There may be the profound fear that, if a good emotional contact is allowed and acknowledged without being denigrated, it carries the threat of a dependent relationship being formed with an other who is not under one's direct control. Also many people who turn to addiction do so in order to soothe the terrible negative internalisations resulting from childhood abuse.

An important result of the deficit in positive internalisations is that there is insufficient identification with helpful parental care or control, leaving the personality depleted in its capacity for self-care or benign conscience. Furthermore, as a consequence of splitting, addicts are frequently in one extreme emotional stance or another. They may be governed by a harsh and judgmental attitude to themselves that allows no mediation and can lead to destructive attacks on the self and/or others by direct or indirect means; or the picture can be one of delinquency or corrupting subversion, as depicted in the vignette above about Linda. In this case the impression is that the punitive and demanding side of the addict is so unbearable that it must be projected onto outside figures of authority who are then angrily or triumphantly dismissed, but at the same time invited to retaliate.

The need for self-punishment is evident in many of the actions taken by addicts but most centrally in their masochistic relationship with the drug and the suffering involved in the lifestyle that they are subjected to by the addiction. When the self-punitive aspect of the personality takes over in an unmodified way, the drug can be ingested on the basis of sadistic destructive impulses and persecutory guilt and anxiety. In this state the drug is felt to be a bad substance, incorporation of which symbolises an identification with damaging objects. In this state of mind the pharmaco-toxic effect is to increase the omnipotent power of the destructive drive, and addicts may give themselves over to unmediated destructiveness directed against external and internal relationships and themselves. In this extreme state, all hope, progress and insight seem to be lost.

For example, Brenda drank heavily during her unhappy marriage and when divorced lost custody of her children. Although she rarely drinks now, she feels unable either to discuss visits with her ex-husband or to pursue regulated legal access in the courts. She feels bound to lose because her husband and in-laws are presented as a powerful, criminal gang. Despite her daughter's affection, she states that even if she won her claim to access the children would reject her. Onto her external life situation is projected an omnipotently destructive internal gang of accusers who allow no recognition of change or possibility of hope. In her mind she is 'the chronic alcoholic' mother who can never be forgiven. The drinking when it occurs is calculated to confirm this picture of utter hopelessness, with her only binge in more than a year leaving her having to ring her ex-husband while drunk to cancel a long-planned day trip with her children to a funfair. These sadistic attacks on herself at times reach literally suicidal proportions, with all hope and will to try to bring about change projected into the group and staff and then thwarted by self-destructive actions.

## Using drugs depressively

Drugs can also be used depressively, when the psychic meaning is experienced as the concrete incorporation of a damaged object with unconscious guilt as a prime motivator. Fundamentally, it is the frustrating early mother that has been attacked inside the self, leading to a vicious circle of hatred and consequent persecutory guilt. This self-destructive unconscious determinant can lead to masochistic choices in lieu of facing a guilt, which, while unexamined, is felt to be omnipotent.

Denise and Jack are two of our group members whose drug use seems to be based on underlying depressive anxieties. Denise grew up with her ambivalently regarded single mother, who had a succession of partners. She was sexually abused by more than one man, including her stepfather. She had abused drugs and alcohol since her early teens. Psychologically, her drug use seemed to be linked to repeated involvements in unbearable or abusive situations. One such situation was her job as a nurse in a hospice for terminally ill patients. She was often the one to administer the final injection of morphine. She became an intravenous drug user during this period, using the same drugs that she was administering. The underlying symbolism of injecting the patients was too close to her murderous feelings towards her neglectful and abusive parents, and her solution was to administer the death-dealing drug to herself.

Jack had angrily turned to drugs and alcohol following the death of his single mother in his adolescence. He acknowledges that he replaced grief with anger and has been unable to mourn adequately. Some years later, he made contact with his father who had left when he was one year old. In the following year, he saw his father a few times before the latter died of an alcohol-related disease. Jack is rarely drug-free and his usage ranges widely. When depressed, he lies in bed overcome by feelings of rage and guilt fundamentally directed towards his dead and abandoning parents. He escapes from this depressed state by drug use, and while intoxicated he manically takes on the entire world and gets involved in many violent situations, particularly with figures of authority.

Jack's inner world was manifest in a session when he announced that his girlfriend's doctor had informed her that she was probably infertile. From his reactions, this news seemed to be emotionally linked to the experience of his mother's death. Angrily he said that his girlfriend was getting a lot of sympathy, but no one seemed to consider what it meant for him. He felt that she was angry with him for his long-standing inadequacy as a partner, and when he tried to speak to her 'there was this dead voice at the end of the phone'. He complained that women always failed him or blamed him. He moved back and forth between feeling omnipotently guilty, as if he was responsible for his girlfriend's infertility (his mother's death), and a dismissive anger that allowed him to be guilt-free.

## Abstinence

We are now in a position to return to the issue of why we did not demand abstinence from our members. First of all, we were concerned that this might tend to set up a view of an externalised authority into which all responsibility for giving up drugs could be projected. We also felt that, as many of our potential members were taking powerful prescribed psychoactive medication such as antidepressants, tranquillisers and methadone, such a demand might feed into their propensity to split by allowing us to be represented as being at odds with other professionals. This in turn might be used to support a split view of authority as either harshly judgmental and prohibitive or as corrupt and hypocritically self-serving – 'our prescribed drugs are good, your illegal drugs are bad' – thus justifying opposition and covert subversion.

We also hoped that, by shifting the focus from 'are you or aren't you using?' to the underlying feelings involved, we might sidestep a moralistic success/failure ethic, which can easily become punitive in its operation and give rise to bitterness and disappointment when time clean is not found automatically to equate to happiness. It might also reduce the potential for destructive triumph over a 'stupid' staff who fail even to realise that someone is using. Our stance was therefore that if a member's drug use either interfered directly with the process of a meeting or gave rise to difficult feelings in other members that was not a problem for the staff alone to address; it was a problem for the group and all its members.

Some of our reasons for opting for group rather than individual psychotherapy for this client group also reflect our belief that the characteristic disturbance of the addict's early object relations and the typical defences adopted will make for particularly severe difficulties in the transference. We hoped that by working in a group we might be able to avoid all of these transference difficulties being focused in one relationship, because there would be multiple transference figures on offer: the staff, both as a couple and as individuals, the institution in which the group meets, the group itself and the individual group members. In addition, patients in a group are constantly moving and being moved between different subgroups, roles, memberships and allegiances. We felt that all of this was likely to reduce the intensity and chronicness of the splitting in the transference and hence also the chances of a patient (or therapist) becoming entrenched in any one position. We also hoped that the movement between positions would support members in continuing to make use of their (at times considerable) functional capacities, making pathological dependency less likely while allowing healthy dependency to be fostered.

Finally, we believed that addicts do not tend to experience objects as being reliable and hence are continuously searching for an ideal reliable object (in fact, this is one of the common views of drugs). We hoped that the group itself might come to be seen as reliable, but with its reliability experienced more realistically as dependent on members' own care for the group, rather than being attributed to an omnipotent staff who could be idealised or, when things go wrong, utterly denigrated.

The extent of such idealisation, and the effect of its collapse, is well illustrated by David. A founder member of the group, for two and a half years he did not miss a single meeting, idealising himself and the group in this, because even the staff took some days off. When the announcement was made of Vince's death, David leapt to his feet and shouted, 'We have failed, James!' After this, though he remained a member for a further two years, he never really settled into regular attendance again. Jack described the same speedy collapse of belief in the goodness of the group after he had been left alone in the waiting room for a few minutes before any other members arrived. He told us that he had thought, 'Nobody's coming to the group because it is so unworthy – does that make me unworthy for coming? – I'm not coming next week.'

In this, Jack is showing us how unreliable the group is for these patients and how likely to abandon you upon the instant. This was powerfully enacted in one of our groups over a period of weeks leading up to a two-week summer holiday, when only two or at most three members would arrive for each meeting. Each member would complain vehemently about the unreliability of the absent members but would then themselves miss the group without compunction in following weeks. It seemed better to identify with the aggressive abandoner than to be contaminated with the unworthiness of the abandoned and denigrated group, which only the staff are left to keep reliable and valued.

On another occasion, the splitting between the idealised and the denigrated group as we approached a one-week break was of a different, though even more dramatic, kind. We had been aware for some time that members were hanging around chatting to each other on the doorstep after meetings and had addressed this in the group. In the penultimate meeting before the break, however, Anne came in and very dramatically revealed a web of external contacts of which we knew nothing. She had been employing not only Jeff but also his wife and daughter to do various chores for her; Clive had given two Valium to Jeff on the doorstep after last week's meeting; members had been going straight from the group to the pub together. Having revealed all this, Anne exploded out of the room, saying that she was never coming back because she could never trust other members again. The idealised nature of the outside group, which narcissistically owed nothing to staff, was entirely evident from the reported topics of conversation in the pub: 'magic and angels'. The corresponding denigration of the real group is only too obvious.

Having set out something of the reasoning at the planning stage that led us to set up our groups in particular ways, we will now turn to our actual experiences in these groups and the developments in our thinking that have followed.

## Two populations

With hindsight, we feel that we can now differentiate two broadly distinct populations of members who passed through our groups: those who over time made discernible and sustained progress, all of whom eventually left on a reasonably positive basis, and those for whom progress, though it might be evident at times, was never sustained. These people became entrenched members, never leaving except in the most catastrophic circumstances. In the discussion that follows, we will refer to these two types as, respectively, 'the improvers' and 'the entrenched'. We are not suggesting that this distinction between individuals is hard and fast. Each member was capable of functioning in both ways at different times, and the culture of the group could tend to promote either mode of functioning depending on its current state. We are, however, saying that in any individual one mode may tend to predominate and that this tendency can be so marked as to justify characterising that person as one type or the other, at least for discussion purposes here.

We believe that for improvers, group therapy is the treatment of choice for all of the reasons already discussed as having guided our initially opting for a group. Groups also have a role to play for the entrenched, but both the treatment aims and the organisation of the group will need to be different. Because we were not clear enough about this distinction when we set up our first group, we did not put in place the structures that might have enabled us to control certain pathological elements as they emerged, and this led to considerable difficulties for group functioning in the longer term.

From a practical point of view, the greatest problem arose from a process that we came to call 'silting up'. Because improvers move on and entrenched do not, over time groups come increasingly to be composed only of the entrenched. Furthermore, this proved a vicious circle, because as the group membership became more entrenched so the atmosphere became more hopeless and delinquent. Thus not only were potential new members pushed towards entrenched functioning, but also it tended to be only those who were already towards that end of the spectrum who chose to remain. Hence these propensities were reinforced throughout the whole group and the cycle continued.

It was our growing belief that the group culture had become irrecoverably entrenched and that this was actively harmful and dangerous to members, which led us eventually to bring our first group to a close. Thus the issue of distinguishing the improver from the entrenched is not simply an interesting theoretical construct, it has profound practical implications, and it will be a very important part of the staff's function to monitor and manage it. Ideally, this begins at the assessment phase so that attempts can be made to maintain an appropriate balance as new members are introduced, but inevitably it will also have to be an ongoing process in which this aspect of the group's current state is kept under constant review in an effort to prevent the culture tipping too far towards the entrenched.

Just as we would not claim that the distinction we are discussing is hard and fast, nor would we claim that we have hard-and-fast criteria for distinguishing between the two types we are postulating. However, it seems to us that the differentiation is broadly congruent with the distinction between 'honest' and 'dishonest'. We do not use these terms to imply a moral judgement but simply as descriptions of characteristic ways of relating to the self and to others. In the context of the group, these different ways of relating often manifested themselves in the ways in which the group and the staff were both experienced and treated. The central question seemed to be whether staff were seen as fundamentally helpful, and therefore to be told honestly what was going on, or whether we were primarily regarded as inquisitors, and often corrupt inquisitors at that, from whom the truth was therefore to be hidden.

## Disclosure of drug use

Perhaps the prototypical issue was how instances of drug use were brought into the group. An improver would bring their drug use forward spontaneously and promptly; one would not suddenly discover that it had been going on secretly for weeks or months. With the entrenched, by contrast, one would often hear about it in passing – 'Oh yeah, didn't I mention that?' – or it would come out in a flood when it could be hidden no longer because the sense of shame had become unbearable. In other words, the entrenched enacted their view of authority as either being stupid and to be hoodwinked and triumphed over or as being harshly judgmental and likely to mete out richly deserved punishment. For the improvers, both group and staff were seen as fundamentally benign potential sources of help; so there was no point in keeping drug use secret and no need to remain silent out of fear of rejection or punishment.

Connected to this was the question of how giving up drugs was viewed. It was noticeable that, for an entrenched member, lip service might be paid to this idea, but very soon some equivocation would creep in: they would just go on using a bit. This could take two forms: either they would intend to go on using the drug that was the major problem for them but in a controlled way (this was most common in relation to alcohol) or they would propose to cut out the use of one drug, which at that point was seen as the problem, but intend to go on with another, the use of which they would claim to be able to control even when past experience showed they could not.

Improvers were typically more honest with themselves in assessing the risk to them of particular drugs. However regretfully, they acknowledged without equivocation that there were certain drugs that they had to give up, but they might also accurately know that alcohol was not a problem for them and continue to drink moderately. If prescribed medication, such as antidepressants, they would consider whether or not to try it in much the same way as other patients without identified drug problems

For the entrenched, prescribed psychoactive medication often presents significant problems, particularly if, like Valium or methadone, it has what one might loosely call mood-altering properties. They may quickly come to feel that they cannot do without it (that is, they are addicted). (Thus we have come to regard it as prognostic of an entrenched stance for any patient to be on a maintenance methadone programme rather than a fairly rapidly reducing one.) At such times, addicts may feel themselves to be in the care of a collusive carer/helper who knows that nothing can be expected of them, and as such they will swallow anything they are given. Alternatively, they may become very angry with the professional who is seemingly (and recklessly) pushing them into using drugs, thus projecting the tendency to drug use onto a cruel external authority who neither understands them nor has their interest at heart. Such figures are often felt to have their own corrupt agenda in promoting the drug use. In both states, however, the drug use is the responsibility of some external prescriber rather than a problem for the user to struggle with.

Improvers who find that they are not as successful as expected in controlling their use of a drug (whether prescribed, legal or illegal) will quickly bring this back to the group for discussion and will struggle, albeit reluctantly, to give up this drug too. The entrenched, however, may try to conceal what has happened, assert that next time it will be different or say that they have seen the light and will simply never do it again, without acknowledging how difficult this may prove. In summary, improvers tend to see what is involved in change realistically, whereas for the entrenched it is either a magical transformation or impossible. Once again, the improver's relationship to reality is more truthful than that of the entrenched.

These differing views of change can be observed in many aspects of a given member's participation in and use of the group. At times, they all know that profound change is difficult to achieve and, at least initially, very fragile. All of them, therefore, are capable of being moved to hear of another member's difficulties and setbacks and of then offering sympathetic support and perhaps also worthwhile advice. Sometimes, however, members will reinforce the delinquent tendency, perhaps by laughing at the account (see the vignette on p. 101 above) or by supporting a view that it was somebody else who forced the member into their delinquent behaviour. A frequent reaction is to say nothing in response to a very distressing communication that might have echoes for themselves but instead turn with narcissistic disregard to another topic, leaving the original speaker alone with their despair and self-reproach.

### Distinction between improvers and the entrenched

Though each member of the group is likely to manifest all of these responses at one time or another, there is a distinction to be drawn between the improvers and the entrenched. With the improvers, their helpful tendencies predominate while the delinquent or despairing tendencies can be mastered fairly quickly, either by the patient alone or in response to the staff's or the group's efforts to draw attention to what seems to be going on. For the entrenched, however, it seems that the sustained contact with psychic pain that is necessary if one is to be able to support oneself, let alone offer help to someone else in difficulty, proves unbearable, and thus they quickly slide back into one or another of the defensive postures that are so familiar in relation to their own abuse. It is as if the improver has a firm-enough footing on the bank to be able to reach out to a drowning colleague and really try to pull them out of the water. If they start to fall back into the water themselves, they can either regain their own footing or, when someone else grabs their coat tails, they can be pulled back onto firm ground. The entrenched member may also try to reach out to the drowning man, but their own place on the bank is so insecure that they soon fall back into the water too, or feel that they have no alternative but to turn their back and leave the victim to drown. Though this image may seem fanciful, it does capture something of the sense of constant collapse – one step forward two steps back – that can be so hard to bear in working with a group in the entrenched mode. At such times, any faith in the possibility of receiving help from another that does remain in the group is probably left for the staff to hang onto as best they can.

Thus we are suggesting that the distinction between the improver and the entrenched has something to do with the expectations that each harbours about the capacity and willingness of others to offer an effective, helpful and benign response to their desperate need. We are also implying that this is related to an orientation towards honesty or dishonesty. This is, in effect, a simplified restatement of much of what was argued in the theoretical discussion at the beginning of this chapter about the quality and nature of the internalisations and the capacity to find a good object. Psychoanalytic theory would lead us to anticipate that these fundamental expectations of others (which in a very simplified form is what is really meant by 'object relations') will be enacted, via the transference, in relation to people and things encountered in the subject's everyday life, including in this case both the group itself and the staff members working in it.

We can better illustrate this by returning to David's cry of 'We have failed, James!' when given the horrible news of Vince's unexpected and unexplained death. Admittedly, there are elements both of idealisation and omnipotence revealed by this response, but the fundamental expectation is of a group that could and should be capable of helping, and that 'we', staff and patients together, share in creating and maintaining it. Thus even such a terrible event as this can (and must) be acknowledged and thought about directly rather than denied, hidden or blamed on others. In that sense it is treated honestly, and we would argue that this is bearable exactly because the group is felt fundamentally to be helpful, even in the face of this awful setback. This was not just a flash in the pan for David. Over succeeding months he continued to return to Vince's death, to try to point out times when he felt it was affecting the group's current functioning and to try to draw lessons from it. All of this behaviour is characteristic of the improver stance, and, though David never did fully settle back into the group after this tragedy, he was still one of the members who made significant therapeutic gains overall.

David's participation was not always positive, however. At one point, over a three-week summer holiday, he and a female member, Amanda, had a brief sexual relationship (in direct contravention of one of the four rules of the group). In accordance with the rule, however, these facts were shared with the group on our return from holiday and thus over the next few weeks we were able to follow through the highly negative ramifications for the group of what had happened. David was able to recognise this, to feel appropriate guilt and regret and to accept the discovery that the rule had been imposed by staff for the protection of the group that he valued because they knew better, not as an exercise of arbitrary and vindictive authority. In other words, his fundamentally benign view of appropriate authority allowed him to feel depressive guilt and thus to learn from the experience in a way that could lead to change.

By contrast, Jeff was not able to learn from these same experiences. He was one of the members who had been most adversely affected by the fallout from David's relationship with Amanda and, as we described above, he was also centrally involved in the doorstep group which was exposed by Anne and used as the reason for her explosive departure. Staggeringly, despite his genuine shame and remorse when Anne exposed what had been going on, even this and the work on its aftermath did not prevent him continuing to meet secretly with the remnants of the covert social network, with results that were ultimately truly catastrophic for him and his family.

The dishonesty of what went on in the doorstep group was obvious and existed on a number of levels up to and including the overtly criminal. At no point did the staff or the group seem to be seen as helpful – we were stupid and to be triumphed over, we were harshly judgmental, we cruelly and corruptly implemented rules that were in some way for our own benefit not for that of the group or its members. By projection, staff became weak and stupid, while other members became the corrupt figures whose continued presence made it unsafe for Anne to stay in the group. In such circumstances, there is no one to turn to, no place for benign conscience and hence no possibility of learning from experience and changing. One is left truly entrenched.

## Expectations and behaviour

Of course, the atmosphere created in the group by members' expectations and their behaviour also has a very powerful effect on the staff. In situations such as the one we have just described, it is very difficult not to feel stupid and triumphed over, filled with despair and then perhaps angry and punitive. To defend oneself from these feelings there may be a temptation to resort to a manic omnipotence of one's own where nothing the group does can dent one's optimism and hope: one will save them in spite of themselves. Thus one colludes with the wish for a magic answer requiring the patient to bear no frustration and by doing so proves that the truth of what has happened is too unbearable to be contained.

It is to be noticed that in describing the staff positions as 'denigrated and collapsed', 'angry and punitive' and 'omnipotently helpful' we have brought forward again the typical attributes that we postulated for the fragments of the addict's split internal objects. Thus we are suggesting that staff are placed under enormous pressure actually to become the figures of the addict's worldview and thereby to confirm its validity. This is one reason why we strongly advocate working as a couple in such groups:

there is a greater chance that one staff member will be able to observe and interpret what is happening to the other, thus arresting the slide into pathological enactment.

When one member of the staff pair intervenes in this way, however, then once again there is often a distinct difference between the responses of the improver and that of the entrenched member. The entrenched see what is happening as the collapse of a frail and unreliable unit, the staff. They may retreat from this perceived collapse into depression because it bears out a bleak and despairing view of the world. Or they may triumphantly try to play upon and widen the split because a couple is experienced as a gang waiting to attack, and, if they can be manipulated into turning the attack on each other, so much the better. By this behaviour, the entrenched member is constantly attacking and subverting the health of the group and thus weakening that to which they are also looking for help. (As an aside, it seemed that in our groups the entrenched members particularly sought to undermine the female staff member in this way. We would see this as probably being a particular attack upon and denigration of women in the role of feeding mother.)

The improver, by contrast, has faith in and values co-operative working. Thus, when one staff member disagrees with another, they typically attend to what is said and consider it as having to do with the whole group rather than as being a matter simply to do with the state of the staff couple. Improvers may try to widen the breach between the staff couple, or even to create one as David did at the time of Vince's death with his cry of 'We have failed, James!', but for them it is an oedipal battle in which the aim is to displace one member of the parental couple so that they can take their place and become part of a new couple themselves. This acknowledgement of the desirability of the couple is surely a manifestation of a fundamental belief in the existence of a benign and helpful other with whom one wishes to pair. (It can be seen that the distinction we are describing here broadly corresponds to the distinction Melanie Klein draws in *Envy and Gratitude* (1957) between envy and jealousy – in envy the aim is not to acquire possession of that which is envied for oneself but rather to spoil it so that no one can enjoy it. In jealousy the aim is to take something away from another so that one can have it for oneself. In our terms, the entrenched state of mind is usually envious, while that of the improver is more likely to be jealous.)

## Practical implications

Finally, we turn to a brief discussion of what we currently feel may be the practical implications of our distinction between improvers and entrenched for the setting up and running of groups for patients identified as having drug- and alcohol-related problems.

Though we have devoted much space to the discussion of the psychic roots of the distinction we are proposing, it is also clear that the very terminology we have chosen implies a phenomenological distinction as well: the improvers improve. We believe that this improvement has typically been so marked within two to three years of group membership that it is no longer appropriate for these patients to continue to be treated in a group primarily defined around a shared diagnosis of drug or alcohol problems. Indeed, to continue to be held in such a setting may tend to impede further progress. If after two to three years of treatment, however, drugs and alcohol remain a significant problem, this is in itself evidence that the patient is entrenched, by our phenomenological criteria. This does not rule out the possibility of slow change over a longer period, but it does point to a need for a modification of the structure of the group.

Thus for both categories of patient there seems to be an upper limit of between two and three years for treatment in a group of the sort that we have discussed in this chapter. Our current thinking is that the group itself might have an indefinite life but that, within that, individual members would come and go and the maximum stay would be known from the start. Improvers might then be discharged entirely, they might transfer to a general group or they might be offered a period of individual therapy. The entrenched would either be discharged or moved on to a more appropriately structured group.

We have argued that the fundamental difficulty for the entrenched patient has to do with securely establishing a benign internal source of authority, so we suggest that this specialised group should be one in which firmer rules exist around drug use and other delinquent acts, as there will be a long-term need for a benign external authority to support the fragile internal resources. In considering the structure of rules to be imposed, we would still aim to leave as much authority as possible with the group, but it must be more explicit that the staff hold the ultimate responsibility and will act decisively to protect the group from corruption. We would suggest acting more vigorously against behaviour that damages the group than against behaviour that damages the self, and we would also act more decisively against behaviour that has become habitual than against single slips, even if repeated frequently. We would continue to regard the drug abuse as a symptom rather than the fundamental problem, but we would accept more readily than we did before that sometimes the symptoms must be brought under control before you can treat the underlying condition. Above all, we would now recognise more readily that the health of the whole group and the safety of other members may sometimes require that someone be asked to leave even when there seems to be nowhere else for them to go. Perhaps this is the ultimate disabuse that the staff must bear.

# Part 3
# Helping the helpers

# CHAPTER 8

# Psychodynamic aspects of relapse prevention in the treatment of addictive behaviours

SHAMIL WANIGARATNE AND FRANCIS KEANEY

## Introduction

Relapse is the most common outcome of treatment in addiction (Hunt et al 1971). Relapse is a central theme in discourses on addictions, as Gossop (1989) writes 'addiction is a relapsing condition'. These apparently negative outcomes may have contributed to a general pessimism about treatment. The perception of hopelessness that is thus generated influences attitudes in many spheres, for example taking on addicted individuals for treatment, the exploration and development of new treatment approaches and decisions of professionals from various disciplines not to work in the area. A further example is that of general practitioners who refuse to work in shared care arrangements with the least damaged drug misusers. The view that the majority of addicted individuals are 'untreatable', taken by many analysts, may also be a reflection of this pessimistic outlook. Some psychotherapy departments operate a policy requiring clients to be substance-free for a set period of time of up to two years, thus discouraging the idea that earlier psychological interventions, or even assessment, might be possible. It can be argued that this stance has had its influence beyond the psychodynamic world to the world of psychological therapies in general, which have adopted a narrow view of the scope of psychological treatment in the area.

Treatment approaches, such as relapse prevention (Marlatt and Gordon 1985), motivational interviewing (Miller and Rollnick 1991), cognitive therapy (Beck et al 1993) and brief-solution focused therapy (Cade and O'Hanlon 1993), have, however, contributed to a widening of the scope of psychological work in the treatment of addiction. Such approaches have also helped to integrate different treatment perspectives and functioned as bridges between diverse conceptualisations. This chapter aims to explore the cognitive-behavioural approach termed 'relapse prevention' and its relationship with psychodynamic approaches. We will argue for an integrated approach, combining the relapse-prevention approach and psychodynamic therapy within a stepped-care model (Wanigaratne 1997). The chapter will also explore some of the traditional conceptualisations in the psychodynamic world that have may have acted as barriers to the development of theory and practice in this area and will argue for a more practical and holistic (trans-theoretical) approach. Finally, we emphasise the value of psychodynamic supervision for staff applying varied psychological interventions in this field.

## Theoretical perspective

### *The paradox of psychodynamic approaches in addiction treatment*

The failure by analytical theorists and therapists, particularly in Britain, to make a significant contribution to the field of addiction is generally acknowledged. In one review, Hopper (1995), a British psychoanalyst, acknowledges that 'there has been minimal contribution from this perspective to the theoretical and conceptual developments in this field'. On the other hand, in treatment settings, loosely conceived psycho-dynamic theory has had and continues to have a large influence. The fundamental assumption in many treatment settings from the 1960s and 1970s onwards was that the addict would achieve abstinence through a process of substitution with the therapeutic relationship with a drugs worker. Counselling, which became one of the main treatment approaches, was based on loose psychodynamic assumptions but often carried out by individuals with little or no formal training in psychody-namic theory and little skilled supervision. It can be argued that much of this counselling took place under a Rogerian banner with little or no acknowledgement of the underlying psychodynamic processes. Like most other schools of psychotherapy, this Rogerian counselling perspective has thus far had no identifiable theory or model for addictions. However, Carl Rogers' concept of distorted symbolisation (Rogers 1951) encompasses a broad sweep of ideas that indicate how the individual may acquire attach-ments to behaviours or items which are ultimately destructive to them, despite apparent early benefits to the individual. The psychodynamic processes of, for example, transference, countertransference, projection, projective identification and denial will play a part in the counselling relationship but, in the absence of adequate supervision or a detailed theoretical framework, may account for much of the stuckness and collusion in the work. When unchecked, this can be damaging to both the patient and the counsellor.

There is a further paradox here in that many psychotherapists are reluctant to work with addicted individuals, who are regarded as unusually difficult, while at the same time there has been a burgeoning of interest by psychotherapists in working with borderline personality-disordered patients, despite these patients being seen to be difficult in similar ways. The large overlap in characteristics and symptomatology between these groups has only recently been acknowledged by theorists from a psychoanalytical perspective (De Zulueta 1993, Hopper 1995).

## Theoretical issues and barriers to integration

Early classical psychoanalytic views of addiction were often extrapolations from the treatment of a small number of individuals treated in private psychoanalysis. People like Abraham (1908) and Rado (1933) built on Freud's (1905) libidinal theory, emphasising the satisfaction through drug taking of libidinal (pleasurable) or aggressive drives. The drugs and the practices involved in taking them took on important symbolic meanings associated with early fixations or regressions. It may be recalled that Freud (1905 and 1928) himself speculated a link between addiction and masturbation, viewed as a kind of primary addiction. Misguided or repressed drives are, then, viewed as being at the root of addictions.

Unfortunately, these early views tended to persist and colour later psychoanalytic theory, such as the idea of addiction as being essentially a perversion, even linked to supposed conflicts over homosexuality (Hopper 1995). In many ways Hopper's view transports us back to the early ideas of Freud (1905) and Abraham (1908).

Theoretical view such as these were usually supported by individual case examples and not by any systematic aetiological or epidemiological research. The validity of the observations was seldom questioned by the analytic community of the time. Anecdotal observations translated into a theory have, we suggest, created barriers and an inflexibility of approach that has dogged the psychodyanmic perspective, in relation to substance misuse, particularly in Britain. The theories and rigid stances taken by some analysts have not only acted as a barrier to integrating different treatment approaches but also hampered explorations into understanding the true nature of addiction itself.

However, some more recent analytic views (for example Hopper 1995) have also brought in more salient research ideas, such as the link with traumatic experiences or early situations involving helplessness. Hopper writes that 'the addiction syndrome is also hypothesised to be associated with life trajectories that have occurred within the context of traumatogenic process'. This links the psychodyanmic perspective with an accumulating mass of evidence from other perspectives in psychology, neurochemistry and neurology, associating substance misuse and personality disorders as aspects of a post-traumatic syndrome.

It appears that in the United States a more pragmatic and holistic approach has evolved, adopted by analysts and therapists, which offers the opportunity for greater integration (Khantzian et al 1990, Kaufman 1994, Keller 1996). The new American developments in the area, although maintaining an emphasis on abstinence, have a more here-and-now approach with the emphasis on the working relationship between the addicted individual and the therapist, rather than working on repressed unconscious material (Keller 1996). Rather than being based on the libidinal and regressive aspects of drug taking, such contemporary American analytic views emphasise affect deficits and self-structures responsible for regulating and maintaining self-esteem, self-care and interpersonal relations.

The traditional stance of analytical psychotherapists in insisting that addicted individuals are free from their addiction for a period of up to two years was based on the assumption that the person should be of sufficient ego strength to undertake analytical therapy. There may be some good clinical reasons to support this position, but dogmatic adherence to this stance may prevent a large number of addicted individuals, who wish to resolve their underlying difficulties, from obtaining help.

## Outline of the Marlatt and Gordon model

The cognitive-behavioural model developed by Marlatt and Gordon was an attempt to integrate different theoretical perspectives and diverse treatment approaches (Marlatt and Gordon 1980, Marlatt 1982, Marlatt and Gordon 1985). It is by far the most comprehensive and holistic model available. Conceptually, it integrates conditioning theories, social-learning theory, social psychology, cognitive psychology and Buddhist philosophy. The need to avoid extremes (the middle path) or restore lifestyle imbalance, the move away from the abstinence/relapse dichotomy and the introduction of the concept of lapses or slips are examples of this eastern influence. A conceptual shift that the Marlatt model introduced to the field is to look at relapse as a process that could take place over a long period of time and not to look at it as a simple reflex-like phenomenon.

The key concepts of the cognitive-behavioural model are as follows:

*Once an individual has resolved to change an addictive behaviour or has changed behaviour, this state of affairs holds until he or she encounters a high-risk situation (HRS). High-risk situations are defined as any situation or mood state that would threaten the resolve to maintain change. These are likely to be situations that have been associated with a relapse of an individual. The most common high-risk situations are described as negative mood states, social pressure, interpersonal conflicts, negative physical states and some positive emotional states (Cummings et al 1980). The next stage of the model involves the individual's ability to cope with high-risk situations and the importance of self-efficacy in the process of coping. If the individual copes with the situation, this leads to an increase in self-efficacy and a decreased probability of relapse. The opposite happens if the person does not cope with the situation. According to the model, failure to cope with a high-risk situation leads to a series of cognitive processes, such as dissonance conflict, rule violation effect, positive outcome expectancies of the addictive behaviour and reduced self-efficacy. Together these factors contribute to relapse. The model emphasises that relapse is a process and that the initial indulgence (a slip or lapse) is part of it and in itself is not a relapse. The first part of Marlatt and Gordon's (1985) theory outlined above deals primarily with the period immediately following cessation or an intentional change in an addictive behaviour. The second part of the theory deals with issues concerning the longer-term maintenance of change. Lifestyle imbalance, where the management of everyday life stressors with adaptive coping mechanisms and strategies is not in place, is seen as a fundamental factor in the failure to maintain change over a long period of time. Lifestyle imbalance gives rise to a number of cognitive processors, such as the problem of immediate gratification (PIG), positive outcome expectancies (POE), denial, rationalisations and seemingly irrelevant decisions (SIDS), which contribute towards increasing the probability of relapse or lead the individual to a high-risk situation.*

Despite the cognitive-behavioural nature of this model, the inclusion of rationalisation and denial, which are undoubtedly derived from psychodynamic understanding, demonstrates the holistic and comprehensive nature of the model. SIDS, which are described as conscious cognitive processes are, arguably, at the crossroads between conscious and unconscious processes. Keller (1996) comments on the similarity of SIDS with psychodynamic processes, such as rationalisation.

Interventions based on this model, or relapse-prevention work, need to contain elements that increase the individual's awareness of the relapse processes, in general and their own pattern in relation to this. Examining the patterns of the individual's previous relapses would help identify the latter. Increasing awareness or insight would also involve looking at the individual's general strengths and weaknesses as well as general coping strategies. Increasing awareness in this context is seen as making individuals more aware of conscious processes (taking people off autopilot). However, a downplaying of the importance of unconscious processes in increasing awareness can be seen as a serious limitation of the model. In reality, becoming aware of or understanding one's patterns of behaviour invariably involves unravelling unconscious processes, whether or not this is the focus of the work. This important omission can be seen as another example of the polarity of approach where one perspective denies the existence of the other rather than taking an integrative view. Relapse prevention requires the development of specific coping strategies to deal with high-risk situations, such as skills training, and more global coping strategies that would address issues of lifestyle imbalance and covert antecedents of relapse. A good relapse-prevention programme would include all the above elements and instil in an individual a sense of preparedness and confidence similar to that of individuals who have undergone a good programme of 'fire training' or 'fire drill' (Wanigaratne et al 1990). The global coping strategies described in this model may indeed include psychotherapy or a therapeutic relationship as well as attending self-help (for example Twelve-step) groups.

*An integrative stepped-care approach: a solution to the problem*

A possible solution to the problems both in delivering relapse prevention and in the conceptual sphere raised in this chapter is to adopt a holistic and integrative approach to addiction treatment. The stepped-care model outlined below for the treatment of heroin use (Wanigaratne 1997) not only offers a solution to many of the problems raised in the area of relapse prevention but also has the promise of placing in context most of the interventions used in the treatment of addictive behaviours. The concepts of matching treatments or stepped care are not new. Nevertheless, attempts at truly integrating the existing models and treatment options in addictions are rare. The stepped-care approach can be seen as an arrangement of addiction treatment according to the Orford (1991) non-neuroadaptational model of addiction. The Orford model suggests that addictions are maintained by three categories of factors, which are termed primary, secondary and tertiary, which are independent of psychobio-logical factors and may act simultaneously. Primary factors are concerned with reward or positive outcome expectancies of the addiction, secondary factors strengthen the attachment to the addiction and distort objective evaluation (for example rationalisation or denial) and tertiary factors are harm resulting from addictive behaviour (loss of self-respect, relationships and employment) that may contribute to an increase in that behaviour (Orford et al. 1996). Interventions may need to untangle these factors and target them individually in a hierarchical fashion.

The stepped-care model integrates the Orford (1991) model, Prochaska et al's (1992) model of change, the Marlatt and Gordon (1985) model, motivational interviewing (Miller and Rollnick 1991) and psychotherapeutic approaches, among others. In doing so, it resolves many of the conflicts of applying singular models in treatment. It also parallels a phased-care approach that has recently been suggested in American psychoanalytical literature (Kaufman 1994, Schlesinger and

Robbins 1983). It also should be considered to be in keeping with one of the fundamental principles of psychoanalytical work of a working through (analysis) of elaborate layering of the patient's characteristic ego defences and resistances (Freud 1923, Greenson 1967).

An example of a stepped-care approach for the treatment of an opiate user is illustrated below (Figure 8.1)

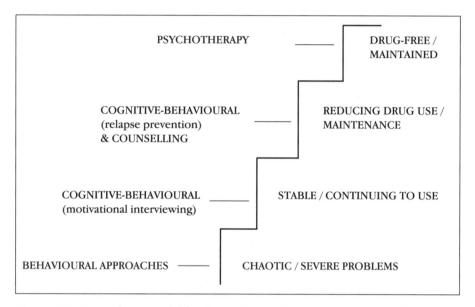

**Figure 8.1:** Stepped-care model for the treatment of substance misuse problems.

### Clinical perspective

*Examples of an integrated approach*

The case of MB

MB was a man in his early forties referred to a community drug service for assessment for methadone substitution treatment. His GP was willing to prescribe methadone with the understanding that this would be a detoxification (reducing regime) and his care shared with the community drug service. He had been using heroin daily for a period of four years as well as cannabis. Prior to becoming dependent on heroin, MB had been dependent on alcohol for a period of ten years and had had a number of admissions for inpatient detoxification. He had not been drinking for five years. The assessment revealed a chaotic lifestyle, with self-neglect and poor accommodation. He also described symptoms of anxiety, agoraphobia and social phobia. Because of his lifestyle and drug-taking, it was difficult to make an assessment of depression. Apart from drug dealers, he had no social network or support system and was virtually socially isolated. He did not report any criminal activity to fund his drug-taking, saying that he used social security money to buy drugs. He had been out of work for over four years. During the assessment, he was not willing to talk about his past or background except to say that he had no contact with his family.

Following his assessment, a contract was drawn up that outlined the conditions of his treatment. The outline of his treatment covered by the contract involved an agreement that he would be prescribed a substitute drug (methadone) at a level that would initially hold him (prevent withdrawals) to the explicit understanding that it would be reduced progressively over a period of time with mutual agreement. He had to abstain from using heroin or any other opiate and produce specimens of urine on request to prove this. He also had to see a keyworker/counsellor at the drug service at regular intervals and behave in a courteous and appropriate manner. The essence of the contract was that, if he failed to keep appointments with his keyworker, produced urine with evidence of opiate use or behaved in an inappropriate manner, his GP would not continue to provide him with a script, and he would be discharged from the drug service.

The first phase of his treatment can be described as a stabilisation phase where he was prescribed a high dose of methadone, as recommended by the community drug service, by his GP. As was the requirement, he saw his keyworker from the drug service for counselling and produced urine specimens on request. Initially, his attendances for keyworker sessions were erratic and his urine samples showed evidence of his continued use of heroin. He was not very forthcoming during his keyworker sessions, with monosyllabic answers to questions, and clearly showed signs of resistance to engaging with the counsellor. He let it be known that all he was interested in was the methadone script.

After a two-month period, the keyworker reviewed his progress with him and informed him that unless real progress was seen it would not be possible to recommend to his GP that his script be continued. At this meeting it was also decided in accordance with the contract that the first reduction of the level of methadone prescribed would be made. During the following four months, MB began to show real signs of stabilisation; his attendance improved and, although he was still using heroin, he was able to disclose this to the keyworker and reported a reduction in the incidence of heroin use. Using the keyworker sessions for practical problem-solving advice, he took the first step towards getting rehoused. He was still reluctant to talk about his past or background.

During the next six months, the most significant development was that he was able to move out of the place he was living in to a modest flat. Shortly after the move, he started reporting periods of abstinence from heroin which was supported by the results of his urinalyses. The level of methadone prescription was gradually reduced to a level that supported this stability – a point beyond which MB was not prepared to reduce at that time. He was also reporting a reduction in self-neglect and indicated that he was eating more. The new flat afforded him the opportunity to isolate himself completely. While this was undoubtedly helping him reduce his drug use, he was having minimum contact with the outside world and his anxiety and phobic symptoms were increasing. It was also clear that the relationship with the keyworker had also changed significantly.

The sessions at this stage were based on the relapse-prevention model and continued to have a problem-solving approach. The changes made or achievements were clearly acknowledged and the sessions focused on an increasing awareness of high-risk situations and ways of coping with them. Goal setting was another feature of the sessions. While avoiding any exploratory work, it was clear that dependence on the relationship was clearly established and was a key factor in his stabilisation. The meetings were fortnightly, and lasted twenty minutes on average. MB started arriving early for these sessions and expressed anxiety when the keyworker had to be away or take annual leave. During this period, the keyworker established that as well as the increasing anxiety symptoms, MB clearly met the criteria for clinical depression. A referral to a psychiatrist or a clinical psychologist attached to the service was discussed with him, and he refused to take up either of these options.

Eighteen months after he had commenced treatment with the service, he had halved his methadone prescription and was not using any street drugs. His self-neglect was significantly reduced, but his psychiatric symptoma-tology was more marked. Around this period he had indicated to his keyworker that he would like to see a psychologist regarding his problems but was anxious that this would mean that he would not continue to see her. Having been assured that any changes to his care would be negotiated, he agreed to see a psychologist for an assessment. The assessment revealed that he was clinically depressed and that his cognitions regarding his self, the world and the future were all of a very negative nature. It was difficult for him to have positive fantasies about the future or what he would like to achieve. It was clear that a reduction in distress was his most immediate goal. He also had severe anxiety problems. He only felt comfortable to go out when it was dark, because he felt extremely self-conscious. He had also altered his lifestyle to that of staying up all night and sleeping all day except the days when he had to pick up his social security payments, collect his methadone and visit the keyworker. He had done his best to engineer that all these events fell on the same day. He was clear that various substances enabled him to cope with life, and, now that he had reduced his substance use to a minimum, he was finding it very difficult to cope in general and with his emotions. He could never see himself being drug free. He was able to give a brief description of his background and his family. He clearly found this difficult.

At the end of the assessment he was told that the psychologist would be happy to offer him a limited number of sessions to focus on his symptoms of depression and anxiety. He was given the rationale of cognitive therapy and given a description of what would be involved. He was told that taking a full history of his life and past was necessary for understanding him and his problems and that this process could be seen as a life review, looking back to set objectives for the future. He was told that he should keep control of what he disclosed when he gave a history and similarly how he used the sessions that were offered to him. It was explained to him that this meant that, if he decided not to continue with the sessions at any stage, it would not jeopardise the continuation of his methadone prescription and that it was his choice to do this work. He was also told that he could continue seeing his keyworker but with a negotiated reduction in frequency. This was to be reviewed after three months.

The next phase of MB's treatment lasted about two years. It started with mainly behavioural interventions of activity scheduling and changing his daily routine. Once he had engaged with the psychologist, the work took a more cognitive flavour, and he kept records of his negative cognitions and succeeded in changing some of them. The rationale of cognitive therapy and the relapse-prevention model were discussed, and the relevance of the work done was reiterated regularly. Taking a detailed history was also commenced after he had engaged in therapy.

MB had an older sister and a younger brother. His father worked in the City and was a distant figure. MB had been very close to his mother, who died of cancer when he was a young teenager. A year after his mother's death, his father remarried. He described absolute hatred towards his stepmother, from the beginning. At eleven, MB had been sent away to boarding school not very far from where they lived. All the step-siblings attended boarding school during the week and went home for the weekends. MB hated school and left soon after his O levels. After doing a few manual jobs locally, he left home at the age of eighteen to work in London. He found a job in a firm of accountants as a trainee. His drinking started around this period, and he had to leave his job after seven years.

He then worked as a motorcycle courier on and off until he met with a severe road traffic accident. Following the accident, his drinking got worse. During the next few years, he received inpatient treatment three times. Since arriving in London, he had taken different drugs from LSD and cocaine to heroin but not in a dependent fashion, although he admitted to being dependent on alcohol during this period. He had had two relationships, the longest of a two-year duration. At the time the history was taken he had had no contact with any member of his family for several years. He did not recall any traumatic incidents in his childhood.

The history was taken over a number of sessions. MB broke down and cried uncontrollably when talking about his mother and her death. He acknowledged that he had not properly grieved his mother's death, and a number of sessions were spent on bereavement work. Deeply held anger with his stepmother and father was the next most salient factor in his emotional life. The feeling that whatever he did he could never please his stepmother and father was paramount. These emotions and the cognitions surrounding these emotions were explored over a number of sessions. During this period, apart from one or two lapses of using heroin, MB's drug use was entirely restricted to the prescribed methadone. His reports were supported by clean urine samples. The level of his methadone prescription was progressively reduced, but he refused to consider coming off. This essentially meant that he had a maintenance prescription.

It was clear that, although the work was taking place within a cognitive-behavioural framework and within a relapse-prevention model, the therapeutic relationship also had a psychodynamic dimension. While analysing the transference was not the central aim of the therapy, it would not be possible to deny that transference was taking place. Working with cognitions involved searching for meaning in order to modify some of the beliefs and assumptions he held, which would also implicate unconscious motivations and interpretations. It was clear that there was an element of dependency present in the patient's relationship with the therapist, and this was partly managed by the frequency of the sessions. Initially, the sessions were weekly but were reduced to fortnightly after some time. Once the improvement in mood and drug use was maintained, the frequency of the meetings was reduced to monthly follow-ups. While cognitive-behavioural work is expected to be time limited, it was felt appropriate to continue seeing MB from a relapse-prevention or maintenance-of-change perspective. Booster sessions or ongoing support seen are important determinants of maintenance of change. It would be foolish to deny the importance of the relationship between the patient and the psychologist as an important factor in the patient's improvement. The continued contact with the patient was seen as therapeutic, while the reduced frequency addressed the dependency issue. It must also be stated that the psychologist received supervision for his work from an analytically trained psychotherapist, and the issues of dependence and continued contact were regularly discussed both from an analytical perspective and from a perspective of clinical judgement. This case, particularly the supervision aspect, illustrates the way that the stepped-care model and the relapse-prevention approach can act as a bridge between the psychodynamic approach and the other approaches in this area. During this phase of his treatment, MB overcame his anxiety problems and depression to the extent that he started work again, made contact with a number of members of his family and made plans to go to college. Towards the end of this period, MB had a setback. Although he did not relapse into drug use, he had a prolonged period where his depression returned. His anxiety symptoms did not return. During this period, he indicated that the work done with the psychologist had made him aware of his thoughts and his patterns of thinking and that he felt that he wanted to get in touch with his emotions. A referral to the psychotherapy department at the local hospital was suggested, and he was keen to take this up.

A referral was made to the psychotherapy department with a summary of his treatment and informing them of his continued methadone prescription. The psychotherapy department responded by offering him an assessment with a psychoanalyst, coinciding with the psychologist leaving the service.

## A relapse-prevention group (RPG)

A common mode for delivery of relapse prevention is the group. These generally take the form of a closed group and run as a structured course of a fixed number of sessions ranging from six to twenty. Sessions are normally weekly and last from one to three hours. There are examples of relapse-prevention groups for longer periods such as a day or a weekend (Wanigaratne et al 1997). We know of a once-monthly RPG now running for several years. Sessions typically are run on themes or topics selected from the key aspects of the Marlatt and Gordon (1985) model, for example sessions on high-risk situations, anxiety management, cognitive errors, lifestyle balance, etc. These generally take the form of an introduction of a topic by a facilitator and a general group discussion on the topic where the members of the group can share their experiences.

In order to ensure that the group understands the model and is exposed to the key elements of it, facilitation in general takes a didactic form. The facilitator is active, being like a teacher or coach following a manual and steering the discussions to achieve the session's objectives and, as a result, some of the more spontaneous group process may be suppressed. Even in the briefest of relapse-prevention courses, it would be futile to deny the existence of group dynamics in the room, which is a further reason to keep psychodynamic ideas in the background of the conductor's mind acting as a guide. Group dynamic aspects of RPG work are largely ignored in the relapse-prevention literature. It is either not considered as relevant or is seen as a by-product of the process, as the work is essentially cognitive-behavioural. Ignoring the psychodynamic aspects of relapse-prevention group work may indeed reduce the potency of this approach and can be taken as another example of the failure to integrate different therapeutic perspective in clinical work. Integration in this area can be achieved by a number of means, for example facilitators receiving supervision for the group work from a group analyst, or receiving some form of group-therapy instruction as part of their training to run relapse-prevention groups. A great deal of work needs to be done from both perspectives to explore the potential for integration in order to achieve the maximum therapeutic benefit for the addicted patient. The following example of a summary of a relapse-prevention group illustrates some of the issues discussed above.

## The group

The relapse-prevention groups we have co-facilitated for problem drinkers contained clients at a variety of stages, who were attempting to adjust to the problems alcohol abuse had caused in their lives. A typical group may contain controlled drinkers, clients on antabuse, newly detoxified clients and recently relapsed long-standing clients.

The groups were structured as follows: in the first ten minutes there was a space for equal airtime for each member mainly to comment on how their week had been and to signal any urgent issues that could be acknowledged and maybe worked through during the current session. The next space was to use some brief solution-focused questions to focus the attention of the group on the present and orientated to both the short-term and long-term future. Then the main topic for that session was discussed, such as high-risk situations. This usually started with a brainstorming session to find out the level of knowledge in the group and to seek examples. There followed some didactic teaching with discussion on how the theory related to the clients' experience and, lastly, some brief homework tasks were assigned.

Groups tend to raise the individual's anxiety and so the facilitators need skill and tact in order to help diminish this anxiety. Being recently detoxified or having experienced a relapse adds to the anxiety. Many found the language used to describe the processes (cues such as booze, alcohol, quantities) affected their internal states and raised their anxiety. For many of the clients it was their first experience of any group process outside of AA or NA and therefore unknown territory. However, the group having a set structure lowered anxiety, and prior to joining there was an extensive induction interview. The group also provided space for silences and reflections, in spite of the time restraints. The therapists tried to maintain awareness of unconscious forces and processes in the groups, such as the ideas influenced by Bion (1961).

The group met for one and a half hours, starting at 11 a.m. and finishing at 12.30 p.m. It was structured as follows:

11.00    Open forum for ten minutes
11.10    Brief focusing exercise
11.25    One of the co-therapists brainstormed with the clients the topic of high-risk situations, introduced RP theory on this and sought examples
11.55    For about half an hour there was discussion on coping with high-risk situations
12.25    For the last five minutes of the meeting, there was a brief relaxation exercise and homework tasks were assigned

Five men and two women attended the group. In the open forum, clients had an equal opportunity to say how their week went and could bring up any urgent issues.

> James said: 'At the weekend, I found myself standing outside an off-licence and remembering how good drinking had been.'
> Mary said: 'I had a stressful week. I have been dry now for five and a half weeks. I feel uptight and find my husband difficult.'
> Patrick spoke about 'thinking about drink and being bored' and 'when out walking, I notice lunatics like myself'.
> Peter said: 'I would like a high without drink or drugs: if I can't drink like a gentleman, I am an alcoholic.'
> Jane spoke about a visit to her solicitor to discuss with her husband access to her children: 'I felt a craving afterwards; I was looking for tension relief.'

The group then brainstormed high-risk situations: phone call to a friend, routine, tiredness, tension, boredom, at parties people who drink, isolation, loneliness, anger, relief, family reunion, being surrounded by booze, airport lounges, feeling in control and attending funerals.
The group then discussed their experiences:

> James said: 'When I went to a wine bar, I did not feel in control. I had one drink – and so on.'

*Mary said: 'I needed space, peace, felt powerless – had four glasses of wine.'*
*Patrick said: 'When I and my wife got back together, we started to have rows – I drowned my feelings in drink.'*
*Peter said: 'Having money in my pocket is a problem.'*
*Jane (who had been abstinent for one year) spoke about her mother coming to visit and of feeling tense and pressured.*
*Ann shared her personal rules with the group. They were: if you have to drink, don't; don't drink to change how you feel; if you must drink, do so in company.*
*The group moved on to discuss ways of coping with high risk situations:*
*James said: 'It's given me food for thought.'*
*Ann said: 'Friends notice when I am bitter and carry resentments. My high-risk situations come with family issues.'*
*Patrick spoke of not doing things automatically and of standing back and seeing things coming like Christmas, birthdays and tax demands.*
*Jane said her plan aimed to 'keep away from drinking companions and to find alternative social companions'.*
*Patrick said again to remember the bad times and the feelings and how much money he had saved. 'I go back to remind myself of a decision not to drink.'*
*Ann mentioned attending AA and of being with people with the same problem.*
*Other coping strategies were discussed.*

### Using psychoanalytical thinking with the above group

Common group dynamics exert themselves in this RPG; processes such as projection, identifications, scapegoating, alliances between patients and attacks on the authority of the co-therapists often in the form of envy. The group's anxiety is lowered by the structure provided but continues to be present. Knowledge of how groups function helps the therapists address these issues.

### The importance of psychoanalytic supervision for individual and group work

Weekly supervision from a consultant psychotherapist for the above group proved invaluable. The communications from the internal world of the patient, the influence of the unconscious, can be easily missed in the hurly-burly of a busy group; so in supervision underlying patterns can be explored. Difficult feelings elicited in the facilitators could also be explored. The supervision, in other words, contains the anxieties of the therapists running the group.

## Conclusion

It is suggested that the cognitive-behavioural approach of relapse prevention placed within a context of stepped care enables the integration of treatment based on diverse theoretical orientations in the area of addictions. Stepped care provides a way forward, as it can act as a framework to stop clinicians falling into the trap of all-or-nothing thinking. We have suggested that some of the more modern analytic approaches have enabled greater understanding and flexibility regarding working with addicted individuals. The work of Krystal (1982) Khantzian (1990), Kaufman (1994) and Keller (1996) can be taken as examples of conceptualisations that are flexible and in keeping with the proposed stepped-care model. The work of Keller in particular bridges relapse-prevention and psychodynamic approaches. An approach that acknowledges the place of cognitive-behavioural interventions, particularly in the early stages of treatment, may also allow for flexibility in the minimum period of sobriety that many analytically orientated therapists stipulate.

A stepped-care approach may also enable therapists to accept the ceilings, or the maximum level of functioning, that their clients achieve. In the area of substance misuse it can be said that, out of 100 assessments, a small minority will go for dynamic psychotherapy, but perhaps more than 50 may be helped by cognitive-behavioural and other therapeutic approaches. The rest may only benefit from physical treatments, substitute prescribing and behavioural approaches. Relapse-prevention and other cognitive-behavioural approaches may help prime individuals to go into more insight-orientated therapies, as was illustrated in the case of MB described above. Integrative approaches, such as relapse prevention, may provide the platform to break down barriers in therapy and research. This could only lead to breakthroughs in techniques and practices that would aid clinicians in their attempts to reduce the distress that addicted individuals experience.

# CHAPTER 9

# In search of a reliable container: staff supervision at a DDU

ROBERT HALE

'In Search of a Reliable Container' was written a year before I finished consulting at a drug dependency unit. It considers the ways in which the addict searches for a container – sometimes in drugs alone and sometimes including the drug clinic. It then considers the stresses on the staff of the unit and the containment that they need.

Let me start with a description.

## The clinic

The clinic at which I consult as a psychoanalyst is part of a large general hospital situated in central London next to a railway terminus. The building is on the outskirts of the hospital and is a temporary prefabricated structure; it has already outlived its intended life. One could say that this reflects the attitudes of the hospital administrators – a degraded speciality. The rest of the hospital, including psychiatry, has a brand-new permanent building opened by the Queen. However, I think it is more complex. It is clear that it is a downgraded speciality in the eyes of the medical world, but perhaps this is what the addict needs, or more specifically what he or she can cope with. More about this later.

It is an outpatient clinic open on weekdays from 9 a.m. to 6 p.m. The staff is made up of eight psychiatric nurses, two doctors, two social workers, one occupational therapist and two secretaries. I go once a week for one hour and have done so for the past thirteen years. Everyone is on first-name terms; often I forget people's surnames. I am invited to the Christmas parties, but I don't go. There is pop music in the waiting room, ashtrays everywhere (smoking is banned in National Health Service institutions) and lots of posters for self-help groups for AIDS, single mothers and benefit entitlements. The patients refer themselves or are referred by an outside doctor or social worker. The majority of the patients are on heroin, which they buy, and which, for the most part, they inject. The clinic is a prescribing clinic. The patients are given a prescription for oral methadone, which they collect from a pharmacy in their own locality. The philosophy is to offer them a reduction programme and weekly supportive psychotherapy in the hope that they will become drug-free model citizens. The reality is often very different. Most of the patients have a long history of addiction with many attempts at withdrawal, sometimes at this clinic, often at another. Often they have been admitted as an inpatient to a detoxification unit elsewhere as a part of the overall programme with support being offered by this clinic after discharge from the inpatient unit.

## Methadone reduction programme

Before a patient is placed on a methadone reduction programme he or she must first have a urine test that detects the different drugs – opiates, barbiturates, benzodiazepines, etc. and registers the level. After a history has been taken the patient is assigned to a keyworker, who negotiates the level of methadone to be prescribed and the time scale over which it will be withdrawn. Overall legal responsibility lies with the medical director. The clinic must notify the Home Office (the Government Department responsible for law and order)[1] of each new patient for whom they are prescribing an opiate substitute. All the prescriptions are signed by doctors and are sent by the clinic by post to the dispensing pharmacy. The patient collects his or her dose each day from the pharmacy.

For many, what I have described will be obvious, boring or already known. For that I apologise. But I have described it in detail for various reasons. First, because some of you will not be familiar with the organisation in England of which the clinic is in many ways typical, although it must be said that the prevalent philosophy in many other clinics is behavioural-cognitive. There are at the most two other psychoanalysts working in drug addiction.

Second, what is offered to the patients is psychoanalytically informed management (or part informed). We are fooling ourselves if we think that we are working analytically within the transference or that any of the normal rules or precepts of analytic psychotherapy are being followed. We are engaged in barter, coercion, support and at times a small amount of thinking with the patient.

---

[1] The legal requirement in the UK for medical practitioners to notify the Addicts Index at the Home Office of any addict they encountered was withdrawn in 1997. It was in force at the time this article was written. This comment has therefore not been removed from the body of the text here (eds.)

Third – and this is my first psychoanalytic point – we believe that, as professionals, we design organisations and programmes to suit the needs of our patients, clients, students or whomever. I think this is an illusion. I think the patient/client designs the system according to his or her unconscious needs and we as professionals in our different roles will, by a process of projective identification, try to meet those needs. This will be true of a hospital, a school, a prison, a residential home for the elderly or a court of law – indeed, any institution. We will construct each institution in hundreds of subtle ways to meet those unconscious needs. The more cohesive the psychopathology of the client, the easier it will be to identify a healthy purpose within the institution – for example a ward in a general hospital or an old people's home. The more fragmented the psychopathology of the client, the greater will be the tendency to splitting within the institution, and the harder it will be to identify a single purpose. The most extreme example of this is a court of law in which we find a prosecutor, a defence lawyer, a judge, a jury, a probation officer, a policeman, a prison officer, a social worker, a witness, a clerk of the court and so on. Each of them believes that they are there because of their professional training, to fulfil the needs of society. This is in part true, but really they are there because they represent parts of the psychological structure of the accused, of which he or she is unaware. The accused needs all those people to be there, or they would not be there. But he or she could not tell you that he or she needs them, because he or she does not know it.

## The role of the drug clinic

Anton Obholzer (Obholzer and Roberts 1994) describes the National Health Service as a defence against the fear of death. I would like to expand this notion and suggest that (1) general hospitals are indeed a defence against death and dying (and loss and physical pain), (2) psychiatric hospitals are a defence against psychological disintegration, madness and to a certain extent hopelessness and (3) courts of law and forensic psychiatric services are a defence against corruption; corruption of the innate sense of justice.

The problem for the drug clinic is that it has elements of all three, and particularly the third, but it masquerades as the second or the first. It is hardly surprising then that the hospital authorities locate it at the periphery and resent spending money on it.

The confusion continues when we look at the names we give to the service: drug use, drug abuse, drug misuse, drug dependency. Each of them is correct, but each represents a different need of the patient. Perhaps we should also add that they represent different needs of the professionals. When we look at drug work, it has very little to do with medicine and less with psychiatry.

Question – why is it a clinic in a hospital?

The most healthy individuals fund and relate to organisations in a defined, organised and mutually beneficial way – examples might be a college in an old, established university or a religious order. Drug addicts are at the opposite end of the spectrum, their purpose is to destroy the structure, to create confusion and conflict, to corrupt – to bring out the worst in an organisation and yet have it survive.

If this is so, how can we relate it to the intrapsychic structure of the addict, his or her use or abuse of drugs, and institutions as a container for his or her anxieties? The next question is what does the institution need for containment and survival itself and, if it is a prescribing clinic, how does it cope with the compromises and contradictions inherent in this policy? I should at this point add that I do not disagree with this policy.

I think that a useful starting point is the 'core complex' described by Mervin Glasser (1982, 1988). In this he describes a situation where the individual is caught between a claustrophobic and agoraphobic fear but with certain qualities. To get too close to the object is to be swallowed up and engulfed and thus to be annihilated. To be left is to be abandoned forever, again to be annihilated. The individual thus lives in a narrow corridor of safety and develops means whereby he or she regulates the distance from his or her objects. Glasser describes this state of affairs with particular reference to sexual perversions where the perversion is used as the regulator. The perversion has the following qualities: (a) it is physically sexually exciting, (b) it confuses erogenous zones and uses parts of the body for purposes other than that for which they were biologically designed, (c) it contravenes a moral code to which the perverts themselves subscribe, (d) the predominant affect is hatred and revenge, which are often masked by sexual excitement (although, as Glasser points out, the ultimate goal is to be reunited with a lost idealised – not ideal – good object), (e) the perversion is the individuals' ultimate defence against negative affect – their vade mecum, which is present consciously or preconsciously and to which they can turn whenever they need (yet even this defence is not totally trustworthy), (f) if the perversion fails as a defence, the individuals have only suicide or murder to protect themselves from total disintegration.

The perversion, in acting as a container, thus has many purposes and qualities and has as a requirement the fact that the body is partly split off from the self and used as a separate object – or part object.

It will not be difficult to see how closely the addict and his drugs parallel the pervert and his or her perversion. (I think it is also legitimate to regard the pervert as a sexual addict.) It is important to recognise that drug addiction is a form of acting out.

Most clearly with the addict one sees the anaesthetic and physically addictive properties of the drug.

## Reasons for attending the clinic

So why does the addict come to the drug clinic? The official message they transmit is that they want help to come off drugs – a methadone-reduction programme. The real reason is, of course, more complex. I think that the addict usually comes when his or her capacity to organise drugs as a defensive structure is seriously threatened. At a superficial level they want a steady supply of drugs, but for this they need to accept a dependency on the clinic and the staff. This is terrifying. They therefore adopt the defence of control by corruption. They score, sell the prescription and tell the clinic that the prescription has been lost or stolen. The addict bites the hand that feeds him or her. It is a compromise dependency. At one level the addict is attempting to destroy hope in the staff and to replace it with cynicism. At another level, he or she is desperately hoping that that hope will not be destroyed, that the object will survive the addict's attacks. But throughout, in a prescribing clinic, there is a compromise. We know our patients lie to us. We attempt to believe them, yet both addict and staff know that there will be lies for a long time into the therapeutic contract. Perhaps the first compromise is to prescribe in the first place – to condone their pathology in order to bribe them to come to the clinic in the hope that a relationship with a therapist can gradually be substituted for a relationship with a drug. Yet, if we do not prescribe, few will seek help.

The danger, however, is that in prescribing we run the risk of creating a system that is as pathological as the addiction itself and that, like the addict, the institution will resist knowledge of itself and thus resist change. It is here that I think my intervention as an analyst has made a contribution in contracting a tendency towards corruption and the destruction of hope and its replacement with cynicism.

## Crisis at the clinic

I first entered this particular system at a point of crisis. The consultant in charge was on the point of retiring. There was a pervading sense of cynicism and disillusionment, and there were suggestions that prescriptions were being sold by members of staff. His assistant was seriously injured in a road traffic accident (not suicidal). The building itself was crumbling and was frequently broken into by addicts.

My ticket of entry was that I was asked to sign the legitimate prescriptions. The senior nurse had to be made aware of the situation. She was, and a major review of the service ensued.

When the assistant returned, he was promoted to being consultant in charge, and I started my weekly discussion group. The focus was and always has been the dynamic meaning of the interaction between the addict and the therapist, as part of the clinic, and to identify the depth of the psychopathology of the patient. The psychoanalyst Harold Bridger (in a personal communication) has pointed out that any new development within an organisation will only survive if there is support from the top of the hierarchy. Throughout my time at the clinic I have had the unfailing and enthusiastic support of the consultant in charge. He has taken part in nearly all the sessions. Occasionally, we have had our own private discussions on the progress of the consultation.

Following an enquiry by the nursing hierarchy, a new system was set up. Nurses would only be allowed to stay in the unit for six months. It was as though the unit was on parole. We focused on the impact that this new contract would have on the therapeutic relationship with patients; as for the impact on the staff, there were two reactions: one of relief at only having to stay six months and one of regret, with many of the staff coming back in their off-duty to ask after their former patients. The staff started to battle with the authorities to stay longer. Eventually, they got back to having permanent staff posts for people who chose to work in the field.

The result was they now had to face the disillusionment of patients who did not get better. They had to alter their perceptions of the purpose of treatment. They could see it now much more as a damage-limitation exercise, but that in itself could be worthwhile. As always we examined in the course of our weekly case presentation the way the patient treated their keyworker/therapist, how they treated the rest of the staff in the unit (as well as outside agencies) and how members of staff felt about one another's reactions to the patients.

**Progress**

Three or four years have passed by now. The staff are staying about two years. They are beginning to enquire about the nature of the patients' inner world. Some of them mention casually that they have sought their own therapy.

An additional doctor is appointed on a permanent basis who has had her own analysis.

Meanwhile, the clinic moves to the larger and better, albeit prefabricated, accommodation, which all are involved in planning. It feels as though some pride is coming into the staff's work.

The preoccupation in the sessions is with the very early stability of mothers and babies. The children are rightly often seen as being at risk. There are many issues around adoption. I do not interpret the clinic's own anxiety about something valuable and fragile being born, yet all are aware of it.

The issue moves on to the patients' destructiveness and their attacks on the therapy and the clinic. Manipulativeness and deception become issues. How can one work with a patient when you don't know if he or she is lying? How do you cope with your own impotence? How do you say no without being punitive? The transference and countertransference can be named and explored.

## Staff development

There is virtually no didactic teaching; the staff find out for themselves – they start a library. Predictably perhaps, it now emerges that three of the staff have enrolled on introductory courses in psychotherapy.

Two of them take me on one side and ask me if I will be a reference for them for further training.

But all does not go so easily. Two of the staff, perhaps as a challenge to me, perhaps in response to the concentration on negative transference, envy and destructiveness in our case discussion, decide to break away. They start a family-therapy project, which changes into a cognitive restructuring programme. They offer the clients hope by concentrating on the positive aspects of their behaviour. Their purpose is to increase the clients' very damaged self-esteem. They see the exploration of negative transference and countertransference as destructive in itself.

By now AIDS is an issue for addicts and the health authority decides to put a needle exchange next to the clinic. I point out via the patients' use/abuse of the two facilities the attack on their therapy and, by implication, the condoning of this by the staff's acceptance of this state of affairs. Always the focus is on the patients. They appeal to the health authority, and the needle exchange is moved.

About three years later, they decide to convene a meeting (at the Tavistock but jointly organised) on the dynamics of drug abuse. Seventy people come from the drug clinics around London with visitors from Rome. Two of the staff – a nurse and a social worker – present papers. It is decided to make it an annual event.

A new problem seems to be surfacing in the case presentations, that of the positive transference, which is perhaps less familiar to the staff. It is likely that they will be less confident in dealing with this than a more overtly negative transference. Later, and more dangerous still, there was discussion of erotic transferences and even erotic countertransference towards some patients. The staff want me to help them understand and deal with such processes and how to differentiate feelings arising from the patient and feelings arising from the staff member. We discuss their pleasure, embarrassment and tendency to make jokes when such material is presented.

Just recently I arrived slightly early to find the director of social work being given a fierce interrogation by the management because she wants to replace a social worker who has left with a shared post. They are furious; they want their own social workers. She leaves with her tail between her legs.

## Summary

How can we understand what has happened?

I think this is an unusual form of consultation. It is not a Balint group. It is not a normal consultation group. It is not a staff sensitivity group. It is not only a case discussion group. I think we have evolved a way of letting the patients tell us how they need the clinic to be and the staff to know more of how they belong within that institution. Problems still abound, but I feel that over the past thirteen years the clinic has matured painfully into a more facilitating environment.

I think my part has been to encourage them to think, to tolerate frustration, disappointment and not knowing. They are struggling to develop a structure that contains and accepts the reality of the patients' pathology but no longer mirrors it or reacts in such a counterproductive way.

I think in many ways the clinic has learned from its patients in the way that Winnicott (1964) describes how a baby may teach a mother how to be a good mother. But, as Winnicott also says, 'Mothers need mothering themselves.' Perhaps I am like that grandparent.

# CHAPTER 10

# Countertransference: our difficulties in the treatment of substance abuse

Luis Rodríguez de la Sierra

We are all possibly aware of the greater attention that patients with problems of drug addiction and alcoholism are receiving at the moment. Perhaps it is appropriate, then, that we should turn our attention to two clearly difficult areas which we have to face with this, until now, largely neglected group: their complicated transference and our no less complicated countertransference.

## The transference relationship

The transference relationship is always an affective one because the analysis is not an intellectual but an emotional process and, for the analysis to proceed, we need what we call rapport. It is only when we make direct contact with the affects by empathy that we can interpret them intelligently and be certain of how the patient is feeling. Accurate empathy is indispensable to sound analysis, and the wisdom we need is a combination of intelligent insight and emotional understanding. We have to register and interpret affect in impulse-object terms, but we also have the further task of analysing the affects themselves. This, of course, applies to all patients, but it is of the utmost importance to bear it in mind when treating the addict who not only deals in a very complex way with his or her feelings but also is capable of provoking disconcerting and confusing feelings in the analyst, who may not always be emotionally ready to deal with them (Rodríguez de la Sierra 1995). The issue of countertransference is therefore perhaps more relevant than ever in the treatment of the drug addict, the drug abuser and the alcoholic.

It is not my intention now to go in depth into the vicissitudes of the concept of countertransference in the history of psychoanalytic thinking. I will satisfy myself with mentioning only what could be called the three main viewpoints of the concept. Before I do that, I would like to clarify that I do not understand countertransference as representing the whole gamut of feelings, attitudes and reactions that an analyst might have about his or her patient. I will restrict the term only to the analyst's *unconscious reactions* to the analysand, particularly to the analysand's own transference. In this respect, Paula Heimann's remarks about the first diagnostic interview with the patient become specially relevant: (1) can the patient be helped by analysis? (2) can they be helped by my analysing them? (Heimann 1959–1960, pp. 155).

**Attitude towards patients**

Some analysts – possibly misunderstanding Freud's recommendations (Freud 1910, 1912, 1913, 1919) – seem to think that the ideal attitude of the analyst towards his or her patient should be an almost inhuman one, devoid of emotions and feelings. The responses of the analyst to his or her patient are thus seen as being due to the arousal of unconscious conflicts by the transference of the patient, conflicts that – if not acknowledged and recognised – become psychological blindspots in the analyst.

Other analysts have the view that all their countertransference responses are imposed on them by the patient.

Paula Heimann (1949–1950, 1959–1960) – and long before her, Helene Deutsch (1926), and Little (1951), Gittelson (1952) and Sandler (1976) – presents the view that countertransference manifestations can be used, in a controlled fashion, for the purpose of the work of analysis. Freud said that the countertransference is 'the result of the patient's influence on [the physician's] unconscious feelings', (Freud 1910) and quite rightly said that they must be recognised and overcome. But it is also true that, when this occurs, it should be used purposefully. In this context, we should also remember his remark that 'everyone possesses in his own unconscious an instrument with which he can interpret the utterances of the unconscious in other people' (Freud 1913).

My own personal understanding of countertransferential phenomena sides with the third of the approaches mentioned above. It goes without saying that I see a personal analysis as a sine qua non condition for the proper and therapeutically useful application of the countertransference to the understanding of the psychopathology of the patients I refer to in this chapter. In addition to it – unfortunately, in some cases, in lieu of a personal analysis – there is also a constant need for clinical supervision, seminars and discussions with other colleagues.

While it is true that the number of confirmed addicts asking for psychoanalytical treatment is small (Yorke 1970), it is also true that, regretfully, the number of psychoanalysts and psychotherapists prepared to accept them for treatment is even smaller (Rodríguez de la Sierra 1995). The reasons for this are numerous and complex, and I will come back to this point later.

Many of the thoughts contained here are personal and may not necessarily be shared by some of my colleagues. They are the result of my professional involvement with this group of patients in the last twenty-five years, during which I have been involved in the assessment and treatment of these patients both in residential and outpatient settings; as a psychiatrist, group therapist and psychoanalyst. My experience has been a varied one, as it has involved my work both in the NHS and as a consultant psychiatrist to organisations specifically dedicated to the care of these patients, as well as experience gained from my private practice as a psychoanalyst. In the NHS and in the specialised organisations, I have been part of a team that worked closely together. The groups in which I have been involved have been mostly slow open groups that I have run and others which I have supervised and which have been both slow open ones and also groups of a predetermined duration.

## Categories of patients

While many of these patients are thought of as suffering from borderline disorders, the reality is more complex. We can see a much greater variety that goes from the neurotic patient to the patient where either the alcoholism or the drug addiction serves the purpose of keeping a psychosis at bay, and to the overtly psychotic person. There is an unfortunate tendency to see these patients as belonging to one and the same category and many erroneous generalisations come out of this misconception. Many times these patients are denied their right to be recognised as psychiatric patients per se as opposed to a sociological phenomenon abandoned to much speculation and theorising. I would like to cite here one such generalisation, an important one to be considered. It is one that Yorke (1970), I realised later, had noticed before me: the tendency to classify the psychopath and the addict as being one and the same. If it is true that addicts may have their fair deal of trouble with the law and become involved in delinquent and criminal acts (in the same way that children, as Anna Freud (1965b) tells us, lie and steal in order to obtain their supplies of sweets), they are not be confused with the psychopath with whom they, by definition, cannot be equated. The psychopath experiences no internal conflict and cannot create one. Instead, they establish a conflict with the outside world that they try to alter by attempting to change the environment both concretely and through the use of magical thinking. The addict does experience an internal conflict and tries to resolve it through the ingestion of substances, which they, unconsciously, use as medicines to 'cure' themselves in that way. This difference is an important one and has to be taken into account for the proper comprehension and management of the two conditions that I will try to illustrate with the following vignettes.

## John

*John, a 15-year-old, the son of divorced parents, had felt abandoned and rejected by his father, whom he had not seen since the age of ten. Undermined by his mother – who constantly criticised him and who found it difficult to tolerate his presence because he reminded her of her ex-husband – John had a very poor self-esteem and had failed disastrously in his studies, in spite of being very intelligent. At school he started mixing with the bad crowd and started experimenting with drugs, first with hashish and afterwards with amphetamines, to which he became addicted, after experiencing for the first time in his life positive feelings of self-esteem. He felt that speed gave him a stronger, more powerful personality which, he thought, helped him to obtain his friends' admiration. In the course of treatment, he was able to acknowledge his feelings of inferiority and how he took drugs in order to improve himself and feel, in his own words, more normal.*

## Linda

*Linda, a 19-year-old girl who had been sent to a detention centre with a long history of antisocial activities, including shoplifting, handling of stolen goods and vandalism, found herself a patient in an adolescent unit as a result of a probation order. She experienced no remorse over her delinquent activities and was convinced she had been caught only as a result of not being clever enough. The family history revealed an early life of emotional deprivation with a sadomasochistic relationship with a mother who had never helped her to master her environment, leaving her with the conviction that she could only conquer the environment by altering it if she had special powers.*

*Magical thinking permeated her mental life, and she only responded to treatment whenever she felt that she was in the presence of a more powerful and clever therapist whose magic she could steal.*

## Neglected group of patients

The understanding and treatment of the delinquent and psychopathic patient have been dealt with by other authors (Aichhorn 1935, Hoffer 1949, Eissler 1950), and I do not intend to enlarge any further on a theme that is beyond the scope of this chapter. However, I would like to end by mentioning another frequently observed difference: the affect of the addict is usually a troubled and depressed one; there is none of the defiance, self-confidence and open aggressiveness of the psychopath in them unless, obviously, under the effects of drugs or alcohol.

Very often this group of patients is dismissed as unmanageable and untreatable and left to the care of organisations and people who may soon find themselves overwhelmed by the enormous challenge that the addict and the alcoholic present, but it is my personal opinion that this neglected group of patients – who may be seen by some as impossibly difficult – is as entitled to ask for help, and obtain it, as anyone else.

Many of the people who suffer from a compulsion to use drugs and alcohol do so because of a powerful psychological dependency that pushes them towards drugs and alcohol in order to avoid, regulate or run away from feelings which can be extremely painful and distressing. An additional complication is the great difficulty (or impossibility at times) to distinguish between symptoms resulting from pharmacotoxic effects and the underlying pathology. The question of physical dependence has to be borne in mind when thinking about those so seriously addicted to their drugs that their craving for the drug requires immediate gratification and becomes the major priority in their lives. Because problems of substance abuse can occur at any level of society and affect any kind of socio-economic group, it becomes extremely important for the therapist to assess how close or remote the patient's problems are to his or her own problems.

However harmful the drug may be felt to be, it has a necessary function, since the addict feels there is something bad inside them (anxiety, guilt, perversion, psychosis, etc.) and uses the drug as if it were a medicine to anaesthetise or destroy the badness, to 'cure' themselves. Drug abusers are self-medicators who desperately and in vain try to deal with powerful, intense and disturbing inner experiences that threaten to overwhelm them. Often, these patients crave to be united with an ideal object. Frequently, when they develop an initially intense positive transference reaction when meeting an analyst, this is linked with the unconscious fantasy that this ideal object has finally been found. Alas, the conflict experienced by the addict is that at the same time, they dread that union with the object and feel persecuted by it. They then become addicted to acting out the drama of fantasy introjection and separation from the drug, a relationship to the drug which is confused and bound up with the relationship to the analyst. The enormous aggression involved, the envy of the object, the great demand for the gratification of very primitive oral fantasies, might create in the analyst fears of being devoured or destroyed, and one often becomes concerned with giving too much or too little. The therapists who become preoccupied with giving too much or too little find themselves in a dangerous situation; they experience difficulties in setting boundaries and in containing both their anxiety and that of the patient. Very often the therapist retreats to his or her containing role and unnecessarily prescribes either too much, too little or no medication, irrespective of the patient's realistic needs.

Many of the initial reactions of the patient are of such an intense and threatening quality that the therapist becomes overwhelmed and unwilling to respond positively to what is experienced by the analyst as a dangerous and threatening storm coming from within the patient. It is here where, in addition to an accurate understanding of the addictive psychopathology and a great deal of empathy on the side of the analyst, one must be prepared to adopt the role of the indestructible object if one is to meet the great challenge the addict presents us with.

## Alan

*Alan, a 19-year-old heroin addict, the only child of an apparently normal family, good-looking, intelligent and a good athlete, concealed a violent nature under a pleasant and polite façade. Like many of his kind, his self-esteem was rather low. Previous to his drug-taking, he had a history of outbursts of violence in school manifested in the bullying of other children and, occasionally, gang fights and vandalism. His eccentricities, shyness and outbursts of violence had made him a rather isolated youth with no friends at school. He hated his violence and immediately conveyed to me that heroin made him feel much more peaceful, more at ease with himself, less aggressive and less violent. He felt less paranoid and more willing to make friends with others. He felt better liked, particularly by the trendy youths who were experimenting with soft drugs and also cannabis and even heroin as something glamorous, attractive and daring.*

*Alan was in analysis with me for four years. After an initial period, when I felt he was trying to frighten me with accounts of indiscriminate and dangerous drug-taking, he seemed to feel reassured by my apparent lack of response. As the working alliance developed, he spoke of the deterioration of all his relationships, starting with his parents who, unable to tolerate the distress to which he submitted them, had ended up by asking him to leave. The analysis of some of the developmental contributions to his self-destructiveness was made possible by his making me into a stronger, saner and safer object than his parents. However, this improvement did not last long, and he went out of his way to make analysis extremely difficult. He would either attack me, saying that my interpretations were stupid and banal, or he would miss sessions constantly. One day he came to see me after a whole week when he had not turned up or telephoned me to cancel. He was surprised to find me in my consulting room and expressed surprise at my persistence when I told him that I would always be there at his times, irrespective of whether he attended his sessions or not. After that session, he started to show some improvement in that he was able to reduce the amount of heroin he was injecting and started to attend more regularly. He was then able to see that his struggle to fight off the treatment was equivalent to his attempts to fight his drug dependence. He eventually left at the end of four years of analysis, having been able to abandon his heroin habit and succeeded in getting into university. He still*

> *keeps in touch with me, and I have seen him once or twice a year during the*
> *last few years. It was clear to me that, in order to gain his trust and if I were to*
> *have any hopes of succeeding with him, I could not accept his destructive*
> *rejection of me and of analysis. At the same time, it was obvious that I should*
> *help him to separate from me and let him take on the responsibility for himself*
> *in making it possible for him to get into university.*

In the transference, Alan displayed his highly ambivalent attitude towards
the drug, now transferred onto me. As a result of his identifying me with
the drug, I would become sometimes an enemy, a persecutor to get rid of.
The message contained in his need to miss sessions was a mixed one: in
one way it was his attempt to free himself from me; on the other hand, he
was also putting me to the test to see whether I would contain and
survive his aggression. To have interpreted the missing of the sessions
only as an attack against me would have been a mistake and would have
lost sight of his need to defend himself against an imaginary attack
coming from me.

### Kevin

> *Kevin, another heroin addict, would report – after missed sessions – dreams of*
> *being persecuted by vampires wanting to destroy him and suck his blood.*

The understanding of this phenomenon and the way in which the analyst
deals with it would greatly influence the possible outcome of these
analyses. Erroneous interpretations based on the analyst's reaction to
feeling massively attacked, might contain a defensive-aggressive
component (on the part of the analyst), which, while possibly gratifying
unconscious masochism connected to guilt on the part of the patient,
could also be an example of what I might – paraphrasing Freud[1] – refer to
as a 'negative countertransferential therapeutic reaction' on the part of the
analyst.

Some of the countertransferential difficulties that the therapist experiences in the treatment of alcoholics and addicts may be the result of some
sort of resistance on the part of the therapist (who may respond in a

---

[1] Freud describes a phenomenon met in some analyses as a type of resistance to cure:
at every point where an advance might be expected in the progress of the treatment,
the patient gets worse instead, as though certain subjects preferred suffering to being
cured. Freud connects this phenomenon with an unconscious sense of guilt inherent
in certain masochistic structures (*The Ego and the Id* 1923). Nowadays psychoanalysts
often employ the expression in a more descriptive way as a designation for any particularly obstinate form of resistance to change met with during the treatment (Laplanche
and Pontalis 1973).

negative way, demonstrating some of their unresolved underlying feelings which are stirred up by this sort of patient). We see this when the analyst finds it difficult to listen with empathy and instead listens to his or her patient mechanically. I am talking about situations where, once the analyst obtains a positive transference from the analysand, he or she responds with interpretations that are off the mark, wrong interpretations which disturb the progress and achievements of the patient and the relationship between them. It is as if we were talking about some sort of negative therapeutic reaction on the part of the analyst whose own unconscious masochism reflects and exaggerates the patient's. I would imagine that here we can also see a reflection of what constitutes one of the pathognomonic symptoms of the addict, namely the oscillations of self-esteem.

## Reluctance on the part of psychoanalysts

There are many other reasons why many psychoanalysts are reluctant to take these patients on. Their impatience and tension intolerance predispose them against the very slow method of analysis. The enormous aggression that these patients act out both against themselves and against the analyst must certainly be one of the reasons which makes them so undesirable. For the treatment to provide any hope of improvement, the relationship to the drug must be transferred to the analyst. The addict oscillates between seeing the drug as a helpful friend and being persecuted by it. In the analysis of these patients we see how they oscillate from idealising us to feeling persecuted by us, thus providing an explanation for their sudden absences, lateness and relapses. All of this is extremely confusing for the analyst, who might experience it as an attack against themselves without taking into account that it is more important to remember that, if the addict is running away from us, it may also be because he or she fears being attacked by us.

In addition to all this, most people who work in the field, in spite of whatever they may say in public lectures or write in their papers, know that the analytic treatment of these patients does not succeed if one insists on a rigid adherence to the classical method. This means that many parameters have to be introduced in the analysis and that the analyst must play a more active role. By parameters I mean those aspects of psychoanalytical technique that can (arguably) be modified to meet the needs of particular classes of patients. Frequency of attendance, length of sessions, degree of management of, and interference in, the patient's life, insistence or not on the use of the couch, are all parameters that may be varied to meet the clinical needs of patients who do not belong to the categories for which classical analytical technique was originally designed (Rycroft 1968).

Even Rosenfeld (1960), who states that there is no need to deviate from the classical method, advised me to introduce certain parameters in the case of a young heroin addict I consulted him about sometimes. When I pointed out to him that his advice seemed to be very different from what he advised in his book, he smiled and told me that, with time and experience, I would learn that sometimes there was a difference between theory and practice. This is a point that many therapists find difficult to accept and – returning to the subject of the countertransference – they feel quite anxious and guilty about some of these parameters and tend to think of them as either acting out on the part of the therapist or, even worse, they attempt to condemn the analyst who thus deviates from the classic, orthodox analytic line, thinking of him or her as either a fool or an ignoramus.

The countertransferential difficulties encountered in the treatment of the addict are not very different from many that we find in the treatment of adolescents. In both cases the therapist is bombarded from every corner with an intensity both in quality and quantity, which, unless well prepared for in advance, one is very much in danger of succumbing to. The most common and easiest way out is to think of the patient as untreatable and reject him or her, even if it is clear that the patient is sufficiently motivated and has some potential for a future psychotherapeutic alliance. In cases like this, a metapsychological assessment is most helpful as one might be able to show to other colleagues areas of psychopathology that can be understood and into which one can help the addict or the alcoholic to gain some insight. The initial rejection of these patients by some therapists does confirm the addict's suspicion of human relationships and all the doubts and negativism about their primary object relationships return to the fore.

## Sean

*Sean was an attractive, intelligent and articulate 26-year-old university student hoping to qualify in one of the helping professions. I saw him for an assessment at one of the places where I work. He specifically required some sort of intensive psychoanalytically oriented treatment. He had a history of drug-taking that went back to his mid-teens. He felt extremely anxious and guilty about it and very much wanted to stop doing it. There were many other aspects of the underlying pathology, but I would only mention here that, when I discussed him with my other colleagues, we all thought we could understand what he was talking about. His use of drugs was an interesting one, and it was not difficult to realise that his use of cocaine represented an attempt to keep depressing feelings at bay, something that also applied to his use of amphetamines. His use of heroin and alcohol, on the other hand, seemed to be very much connected to his problems over sex and aggression. He had spoken about what appeared to be bisexual conflicts, and, although he now had a more or less stable heterosexual relationship, it was quite clear that his homosexual fears were greater than he admitted, and both his use of heroin and alcohol were unconsciously aimed at regulating these bisexual conflicts. We all understood the importance of this, and everybody pointed out how that had to be taken into account, as well as his aggressive and destructive impulses, when trying to understand his use of heroin, particularly when injecting it intravenously. After a long discussion (some of the people at the meeting had experience with this population, others not), where people spoke openly about their countertransferential fears in relation to these patients, a vote was taken, and it was decided to offer this patient some sort of psychotherapeutic help. At that moment, the chairman, quite out of character, decided to exercise his right to vote – something I had never seen him do before. His vote of course changed the whole picture and no treatment could be offered to this patient.*

This clinical vignette illustrates some of the problems for both the patient and the therapist. The rejecting therapist may not always be aware that their rejection, or rather, their rejectiveness, is, unconsciously, their way of being sensitive to the very damaged narcissism of this patient, or in other words to the very low self-esteem and the great fears and anxieties about being accepted. It is a shame that many of these therapists try to justify rather than understand their feelings. It is also a shame that very often they think that, when the patient succeeds in finding a therapist who takes up the challenge, such a therapist has been seduced by the patient and is heading for disaster. This is, of course, a very superficial approach as, if one looks deeper, one becomes aware that the dynamic interaction between therapist and patient is much more complex than that. Hence the need to understand such exchanges. It is true that many times it is a lost war from the beginning, but there is a difference between entering a lost war knowingly and not hoping to win but attempting to do something about it, and foolishly falling into the trap that these patients (alcoholics mostly) present at times to therapists who, narcissistically vulnerable, respond with grandiose and omnipotent ideas of their being the only ones who understand and can help.

## Masochistic tendencies

A common feature in these patients is the highly masochistic way of relating to their external world accompanied, it goes without saying, by a very low self-esteem. These patients, unconsciously, succeed in manipulating the therapist into responding to them in a sadistic way. In recent years, we have seen the influence of a certain confrontational style practised in some institutions modelled along the lines of what is (rightly or wrongly) perceived as rehabilitation programmes imported from North America. Many of these organised therapeutic interventions often offered to the addict and to the alcoholic do exploit, unconsciously, the masochistic tendencies of these patients. In these institutions patients are compelled to acknowledge the futility of their will and are told that in order to improve they must submit their will to a Higher Power (God). Even if it sounds contradictory, I must say that I have been surprised many times with the positive therapeutic effects that the gratification of such masochistic tendencies produces.

### The therapist's views

The therapist's personal values, opinions and attitudes to the addict and the alcoholic need to be acknowledged. This is one of the occasions when the benefits from a personal psychoanalytic or psychotherapeutic experience are clearly seen. Some therapists may be rather intolerant and hostile to addicts and alcoholics in a normal social situation but, through self-analysis, they might be able to use such feelings constructively in the therapeutic situation for the treatment to be effective.

For the less experienced therapist, it must be difficult to accept that one cannot be too ambitious with these patients, as we do not often achieve internal psychic changes of great magnitude. Even in cases where the addiction appears to have been cured, these patients remain rather fragile and very much in need of care and support. The feelings of frustration and their clinging onto the therapist might provoke in the latter a rejection of these patients and a loss of interest in them. Some of these patients may become patients for life in the sense that, once the treatment is finished, they may feel reassured and safer knowing that there is a possibility of resuming contact with the therapist even if it is only by letter once a year. The main problem remains that improvement in the life of some addicts is often more superficial than in other patients and very much related to being able to preserve the good relationship to the object (or analyst), even after treatment, in theory, has ended. This requires special patience and skill on the therapist's part and a capacity to understand and tolerate the great needs and demands of the addict. It is the presence and abundance of such great needs and demands that make it necessary to introduce in the psychoanalytical treatment of the addict the parameters I referred to earlier on. They may at times make the analyst wonder about the feasibility of the treatment. Here I would like to quote Julia Mannheim (1955), who, in her touching account of her analysis of a female addict, illustrates this point well: 'Many analysts agree that in the treatment of borderline cases, severely traumatised at all stages, some modifications, without impairing the neutral reserve of the analyst, are found to be necessary. The panic-stricken anxiety, deriving in part from lack of parental support, must come to a first abatement. Unless they can rely on the analyst in the role of the "ordinary, devoted mother", they behave like traumatised pre-Oedipal infants and their anxiety excess does not permit them to gain insight' (p. 67).

Personal understanding and handling of countertransference problems are absolutely necessary, for such problems can prevent the analyst from recognising the addict's specific needs and conflicts, and from supplying the explanations that may increase the ego strength so as to enable it to deal with the painful affects in their regressed form.

Some therapists with unresolved adolescent conflicts over authority figures may unconsciously collude with the addict. The therapist identifies with the addict's rebelliousness and is seduced by the pseudo-romantic and dramatic presentation of the drug and alcohol abuser. These therapists may also have unresolved unconscious impulsive fantasies that are stirred up and gratified through the patient's acting out. The addict then unconsciously perceives the therapist's unconscious approval of his or her behaviour. This is likely to happen among drug workers in drug addiction units who have not had the benefit of a personal analysis or personal therapy. In such situations, they become identified with the victim aspect of the patient and join forces with them in (a therapeutically needless and misguided) battle against society.

In some therapeutic communities and rehabilitation hostels, it has become fashionable for the treatment of drug and alcohol abusers to be conducted by previous patients. The value of the personal experience that such healthcare professionals may have had with drugs has been magnified to the detriment of the need for their own personal therapy. It is a curious phenomenon as nowhere else in the field of psychiatric or psychotherapeutic treatment is having had the illness a sine qua non condition for treating it. In my experience as a consultant to some of these institutions, only the healthcare professionals who have then gone on to a personal analysis or some kind of psychotherapeutic treatment do not succumb to the pressures of the work. Many of the others, sooner or later, end up relapsing.

The need of the addict to split and provoke envy in the therapist is something that we must be attentive to. Many of them take great delight in telling you how Alcoholics Anonymous or Narcotics Anonymous really disapprove of our work and obviously try to get us to retaliate with some kind of caustic remark. They are often quite surprised when I encourage them to continue attending those meetings because I personally believe they are a great help and I know of the limitations of my analytic or psychotherapeutic work with these patients. In other words, I need friends in the outside world, and that is the role that many of these groups fulfil.

# Part 4
# Community
# psychodynamics

# CHAPTER 11

# Growing up with addiction

MARTIN WEEGMANN

'You brought him up to be a boozer ... Since he
first opened his eyes, he's seen you drinking. Always
a bottle on the bureau in the cheap hotel rooms.'
(Eugene O'Neill, *Long Day's Journey Into Night,* p. 96)

This chapter considers some clinical and research issues around adults
who have grown up with one or two addicted parents, parents suffering
alcohol dependence and/or drug misuse. I begin with a critical discussion
of some of the more popular 'adult children of alcoholics' literature,
followed by some issues arising from scientific research. I then describe
some findings from a clinical survey of the childhood backgrounds of
patients presenting to different clinical services, finishing with several
psychotherapy vignettes to illustrate some individual dynamics.

## Adult children of alcoholics: the movement, the literature

The phenomenal growth of the adult children of alcoholics (ACA)
movement and similar recovery groups, particularly in America, though
spreading elsewhere, is deserving of cultural study. ACA groups were
founded in the 1980s in the US in response to the needs of a neglected
population, providing fellowship and affiliation to people who had grown
up in families ravaged by addiction. Allied to this growth, and usually
sharing the same philosophical base, are co-dependency recovery groups
designed for individuals who might be living with addicted others or who
suffer from involvement in various forms of dysfunctional and controlling
relationships. Co-dependency is sometimes framed as 'relationship
addiction', often understood in the same fashion as alcoholism is understood by AA, as a disease-like process, with recovery seen in terms of the
12 steps of the Minnesota Model.

AlAnon groups, founded during the 1950s for the wives of alcoholics, and AlAteen for teenagers with drinking parents, were the forerunners of these more recent recovery groups. The common ground between these earlier and later groups, however, is the emphasis on reaching out to those others who have been affected by the drinking or drug abuse of someone else, usually a family member. It contains and legitimises the premise that addiction is a shared problem (hence, the use of the expression 'co-dependency' and the notion of alcoholism as a family disease). For every chemical-dependent individual, there will be, so it is argued, several other co-dependents whose fortunes are tied up with the addict. I have heard some advocates of AlAnon argue that the family member is just as sick as the drinker, only is not using alcohol.

One of the most important achievements of these recovery groups has been, it seems to me, to offer an antidote to the shame and isolation which family members frequently endure, reaching as they do into the furthermost regions of familial life damaged by chemical dependence and abuse. AlAnon, for instance, is now a worldwide organisation and in many parts of the UK is the only service available to the spouses of drinkers, with traditional addiction services concentrating exclusively on the needs of the user. Through membership of such groups, affiliation can replace isolation, sharing and identification can dislodge shame and acknowledging the consequences of someone else's addiction on oneself can lead, ultimately, to greater independence and acceptance within one's relationships. Recovery groups can provide a caring environment, offering solace and acceptance to individuals who have frequently encountered blame or invalidation in family life. These elements constitute, I believe, some of the curative and reparative benefits of membership (see Cermack 1989).

Thinking about the spread of ACAs and co-dependency groups, one might hazard the guess that culturally they represent a desire in advanced, liberal societies to locate disadvantaged and obscured minorities and to overcome taboo. An important, landmark book dealing with the subject in the 1960s, for example, referred to such children as the 'forgotten children' (Cork 1969). Attention has been rightly focused on the large size of the population of potentially affected individuals. Perhaps there is in American culture a certain vogue for recovery groups: a disease for everyone, so to speak

While not wanting to underestimate or to decry the support that ACAs and other groups provide, there are nevertheless problems with some of the assumptions they appear to promote. Expressions like 'co-dependency' or 'addiction' itself can easily become reified, catch-all phrases leading to many generalisations about the supposed common experiences of ACAs. Popular books abound, listing numerous symptoms to which ACAs are prone, with such groups leaving us in no doubt that children so affected are, indeed, in the words of the nursery rhyme, like Wednesday's Child: full of woe. And those who do not know it are 'in denial'. Sometimes, the term 'enabling' can also be used as offering an automatic explanation, rather than as a dynamic that is applicable in *some* instances.

In terms of clinicians writing in this area, some authors are closely identified with the spirit of the recovery movements. Kern (1978), for example, writes assertively about supposed 'personality characteristics' of ACAs, the behavioural symptoms they exhibit and the alleged stereotyped roles they adopt in family life: roles like the 'family hero', the 'scapegoat', the 'mascot', the 'adjuster' and so on (see also Wegscheider 1981). One is reminded here of an earlier generation of psychodynamic writers who were apt to make sweeping generalisations about the supposed personalities of the spouses of alcoholics (see the valuable, critical review of the 'disturbed personality theories' by Edwards et al 1973). In Kern's recommendations for treatment, he leaves us in no doubt as to his view that, 'Regardless of age, COAs need to learn the basic facts about alcohol as a drug and alcoholism as disease. This is the entry point, the beginning, which then blends into group and individual treatment'(p. 329).

In a similar vein, Nyman and Cocores (1991), in a contribution on co-addiction and family members, advocate a Minnesota model to confront what is termed the 'enabling system' of addicted families. Enabling concerns denial and the conditions under which the drinking family member is helped, often unwittingly, to continue. 'In general,' they write, 'the psychological and behavioural disturbances exhibited by family members that are a direct result of regular interaction with an addict have been labelled co-dependency or coaddiction' (p. 877). Quite how such direct results are conceptualised is left unclear.

Cermack (1986), who has done much to promote the concept of co-dependence, sees it as a diagnostic entity as well as a psychological concept and has advocated that the problems of the children of alcoholics and ACAs should be regarded as falling within a distinct diagnostic category of the *Diagnostic and Statistical Manual* of the American Psychiatric Association (the American system of psychiatric classification). He argues that the adaptations involved in co-dependency are comparable in most regards to the symptoms of post-traumatic stress disorder.

On the other hand, other writers seem have approached the subject, in my view, with less generalisation or dogmatism, concentrating instead on more subtle processes of adaptation to parental addiction and the problems that can arise when ACAs come into treatment. Beletsis and Brown (1981) suggest a developmental framework for understanding adult children of alcoholics and indicating that 'not every child is affected by the alcoholic parent in the same way. Psychological, social and inter-active factors give rise to a variety of adaptations. The dynamics of the family environment differ depending on such variables as whether one or both parents are alcoholic; the children's ages when alcoholism becomes unmanageable; economic stability; and the availability and use of external support systems' (p. 188). Brown (1997) went on to write an inspiring book on the treatment of ACAs, illustrating the complexity of the issues involved and integrating cognitive theory with psychodynamics, in particular Bowlby's attachment model. Through this she tried to concep-tualise the process in the child of accommodation/assimilation to his or her experiences and the building up of 'internal models', signifying attachment and expectancies towards the parents.

Finally, Vannicelli's (1991) work sensitively explores the countertrans-ference issues, which work with ACAs can stimulate, including the question of how best to conduct professional group therapy with such individuals. However, I am unconvinced that these are all exclusive to such populations, since similar therapeutic difficulties and re-enactments could accompany work with other types of patient.

## Scientific research

A substantial body of scientific research addresses the psychosocial conse-quences on the children of addicts, although it is well known that that there are many methodological and conceptual problems remaining with such investigation. The traditional focus of research has been on alcoholism, with research into the children of drug addicts proportionally less, although there are signs that this is beginning to change, such as the collection edited by Rivinus (1997) and the literature described in Hogan's (1998) excellent review. While not wanting to conduct a review here, I will put forward some general points.

- There are inherent complexities in researching an area often dependent on retrospective accounts, and it is has not been possible to isolate something called the 'effects of addiction' or some pure variable like 'parental alcoholism'. Definitions of addiction – types of drug used, legality versus illegality, maternal versus paternal addiction, the visibility of the addiction to the children, types of behaviour arising from intoxication, dry periods, or how much the family system is organised around the drinking and/or its denial, and so on – may not be consistently or adequately defined. The contribution of factors such as family discord or disintegration, social class, poverty, antisocial lifestyles and alcoholism is notoriously difficult to disentangle. El-Guebaly and Offord (1977), reviewing the offspring of alcoholics, and

Hogan (1998), reviewing the psychological development of children of opiate and cocaine users, have clarified the nature of these and other methodological problems. Like other areas of familial or developmental psychopathology, we are alerted to great complexity facing researchers, a fact which challenges many of the generalisations and causal assumptions claimed in popular literature.

- A detailed differentiation of discriminating themes is essential in the study of such family-related problems, as one faces a complex system, morphologically and over time. Factors such as the nature of the family climate, the adaptation of the non-addicted parent, the influence of siblings, outside support, gender differences, the concurrence of substance misuse with other psychiatric disorders, violence and so on are important to consider. Wilson and Orford's (1978) review, and that of Moos et al (1990), proposes some excellent clarifications of research needs. The nature of the family climate and family discord have, for example, been emphasised as being of greater significance compared with the presence of excessive drinking per se, to use one example. Perhaps research in the area of family addiction has something to learn in this regard from research on other forms of family discord, such as divorce.

- Rutter's (1985) landmark contribution to developmental psychopathology speaks of 'resilience in the face of adversity', and we certainly need to understand more about the nature of resilience in the face of addiction, including that in those many individuals who do not turn to drugs themselves or who, moreover, appear to develop successful coping abilities in adult life, even in the presence of stress as children. What might some of these protective processes be, which help insulate some individuals against stress? Or which allow some children to successfully disengage or to switch off from parental alcoholism? And what makes other individuals, by contrast, seem far more vulnerable or porous to the effects of negative experiences of parental addiction?

- Velleman and Orford (1999), in their important collection of painstaking research reports, emphasise the importance of looking at general community as well as clinical/agency samples when it comes to understanding the impact of alcoholism or the transmission of problems from one generation to another. Adult adjustment will be reflected differently according to one's sample source, as clinicians, by definition, deal with casualties. Community samples, in Velleman and Orford's work, demonstrate quite different patterns of adjustment and coping.

Many of the more careful reviews, therefore, seem to favour a stress-vulnerability model of such family problems with an emphasis on risk factors. There may even be, for some individuals, a paradoxically strengthening element in having to deal with adversity, and, indeed, self-esteem may grow as a result of successful coping and reinforcement by a stable parent or, say, other siblings. However, it is also important to be mindful of the possible construction of what Winnicott (1951) terms the 'false self', which dissimulates underlying deprivation.

Qualifications of complexity aside, I agree wholeheartedly with the recent plea by Rydelius (1997) that familial drink and drug abuse needs to be kept more firmly in mind in psychiatric evaluations as a risk factor and not only addressed when the addiction has already overrun all aspects of healthy family functioning.

• With the exception of the work mentioned earlier, especially that of Brown and Vannicelli, there is a noticeable absence of psychoanalytic literature or reports in the area. This woeful neglect by the psychoanalytic community may mirror a lack of experience with addicts and an unwillingness to engage in thinking about the scale of addiction problems in societal terms. At the same time, different psychodynamic theories could serve as an important source of hypothesis-making for future research in this area.

## Clinical sample

This clinical sample from an audit of the author's practice is intended to offer some insight into reported childhood experiences. The survey consists of assessment information conducted with fifty individuals presenting to a community drug service and fifty individuals presenting to a community alcohol service. This is contrasted with fifty subjects assessed for psychotherapy in an outpatient psychotherapy department, but excluding any presenting with addiction problems. The information thus collated was as a result of ordinary clinical assessment and was not framed or designed as a formal research project. The findings are shown in table 11.1:

1. **Alcoholism** or **alcohol problems or heavy drinking** were identified according to the subject's point of view.
2. **Drug abuse** in a parent meant illegal substances (class A) – no information was obtained regarding, say, the use of benzodiazepines or cannabis in parents.
3. **Gambling** was in the absence of alcohol problems.
4. **Violence** referred to subjects who had been on the receiving end of, or who had witnessed recurrent physical abuse – normally involving a parent, or between the parents and, in some cases, involving siblings.
5. **Abandonment** was defined as a parent who walks out and who, thereafter, disappears from the subject's life, or where there has been only a fleeting or minimal link.
6. **Sexual abuse** meant abuse of various kinds, usually recurrent, both within and outside the family.

**Table 11.1:** Clinical assessment findings

| Incidence of: | Drug users (N = 50) | Alcohol users (N = 50) | Psychotherapy assessments (N = 50) |
|---|---|---|---|
| 1. Alcoholism or alcohol problems | 25 (50%) | 32 (64%) | 5 (10%) |
| *Maternal* | 6 (12%) | 8 (16%) | 2 (4%) |
| *Paternal* | 15 (30%) | 20 (40%) | 3 (6%) |
| *Both parents* | 4 (8%) | 4(8%) | |
| 2. Drug abuse | 2 (4%) | 1 (2%) | |
| 3. Gambling | 2 (4%) | 1 (2%) | |
| 4. Violence | 10 (20%) | 7 (14%) | 8 (16%) |
| 5. Abandonment | 6 (12%) | 7 (14%) | 4 (8%) |
| *Maternal* | 3 (6%) | 1 (2%) | 1 (2%) |
| *Paternal* | 3 (6%) | 6 (12%) | 3 (6%) |
| 6. Sexual abuse | 6 (12%) | 8 (16%) | 5 (10%) |
| 7. Normal/supportive family | 12 (24%) | 10 (20%) | 17 (34%) |

7. **Normal and supportive** meant, from the subject's point of view, a helpful family climate and encouragement.

It must be emphasised that a variety of other problems were described, including emotional neglect, institutional upbringing, family discord, mental illness in a small minority of parents and antisocial problems (criminality), typically in fathers. Also, in the 'normal and supportive' camp some of the more in-depth psychotherapy assessments in particular, did reveal other problematic aspects, such as 'overprotective', 'overcontrolling', 'a lifeless atmosphere', 'overbusy' parents in addition to many helpful experiences. Likewise, when difficult experiences are explored in depth, it is often possible to locate some helpful experiences or an inconsistent rather than wholly bad picture.

**Clinical material**

I have chosen to present eight vignettes of treatment cases, to illustrate some of the differing experiences and individual dynamics of those who have grown up with addiction in the family.

*Sally*

Sally was seen for cognitive therapy, for problems not related to addiction, although she felt that earlier bouts of excessive drinking might have contributed to her difficulties. Her mother had been a heavy drinker who had died of an overdose during the patient's later childhood. She described the rest of the family as being normal. When I tried to explore this history, her anxiety increased, as though she was concerned about what significance I might see in it; in the next session she was able to articulate this in the following way: 'I don't see a link between my problems now and those of the past' and 'therapists are bound to want to dwell on what happened with my mother'. In retrospect, I think she was probably responding to ideas that were forming in my mind about the impact of such an experience. Treatment, in fact, did not concentrate on the past to start with, though at a later stage I did attempt to uncover deeper personal schemas through asking specific questions around the quality of and disruptions to her childhood attachments (see Marrone 1998 for a description of how this can be done).

Her mother figured as a completely unsafe and unpredictable person (with and without drink), who frequently hurled criticisms and insults at the patient. Sally reported feeling disgust towards the mother's drinking and within the family system there were two other helpful and reliable figures, including the father, who appeared to have compensated well in the face of a family tragedy, the overdose.

It is hard to tell with brief treatment whether Sally's view that her past had no bearing on her present-day problems is an accurate one (and/or whether this view needs to be simply held as her understanding rather than prematurely challenged) or whether, as therapy progressed, she was terrified of making a cognitive or affective link to her despised, drinking mother. Subtle interviewing, however, such as the attachment explorations, can help build up a detailed picture of the past with particular instances of experience. John Bowlby (1988a) was surely right to emphasise the importance of actual experiences, and not only fantasy in psychotherapy, and this emphasis might be important in understanding how a parent's addiction may influence the child's coping in subtle ways. It might, for example, be important to ask specific questions about how a parent behaved while intoxicated as well as to address the patient's view of what the parent might have been responding to through their behaviour. Perhaps for Sally, an element of disgust and a familial need to decisively move on following the tragedy had led to an adaptive counteridentification with her mother.

*Bob – a case reported by a supervisee.*

A supervisee reported sessions from a patient who had a drug-abusing father and a mentally unstable mother. The supervisee felt strong concern for his welfare, particularly a fear of what he might do to himself, and alarm at his devil-may-care attitude towards himself. There seemed little sense for the healthcare professional of having a reliable patient present, with many missed appointments and with minimal overt ability to co-operate with the therapist. He frequently abandoned himself to drug binges, using the same type of drug his father had used and during these times saw treatment as an unnecessary limitation on his freedom. Although he could report worry about his actions, this seemed matched by an inability or reluctance to take action, with the supervisee feeling that she carried the anxiety instead. Material from the sessions suggested to me an identification with a very damaged, unstable or even dying container; in fact, 'deadly' was one of the descriptive terms used by the supervisee.

Here, perhaps, we see a patient who had modelled himself on an addicted parent, with another parent who proved unreliable in a different way. The idea of helpfulness or of helpful authority seemed alien to him. His father had never recovered, which may have further handicapped the patient's hope, leading to a seemingly complete capitulation to addiction during the binges.

I believe that the notion of 'double deprivation' (Henry 1974) has good explanatory value for those patients who have experienced early privation and deprivation. In this notion, the individual is handicapped by the original deprivation inflicted on him or her and then further deprived of helpful experiences as a result of the formidable defences that have been built up. It could be even argued that, once drugs have been incorporated into the picture, the therapist can face a kind of 'triple deprivation', as perhaps was the case with Bob. In other words, we face the original depri-vation, the early defences against emotional pain or injury and then a layer of drug abuse as a response by the individual to their emotional pain. All this seriously compromises the ability of the therapist to reach the suffering part of the patient, as appeared to be the case with Bob.

### Charles – a case reported by a supervisee

A counsellor spoke of a drug user whose mother had died of a drug overdose, followed by many subsequent disruptions to child care. The patient, however, retained an idealised picture of the mother as having been the only person who loved him, having no real sense of other attach-ments. One feature of his treatment was his tremendous need to devalue the counsellor, who was seen as incapable of understanding and corrupt. The counsellor found it difficult to be on the receiving end of this dynamic, sometimes wanting to counterattack and at other times to withdraw into an almost passive acceptance of the patient's aggression. Either way, the sessions resembled a power struggle, with the apparent need for a victor.

A dynamic formulation which increasingly suggested itself was that the patient had been exposed to traumatic helplessness and as a result needed to rid himself of any feelings of vulnerability. The counsellor's strength and integrity had to be continually challenged – the counsellor also being, as if often the case with other clients, the only enduring person in his current life.

Here, I would like to draw attention to Bowlby's (1988a) comments about the sad, and underreported, numbers of children who have had to deal with (or even witnessed) a parent's suicide (or overdose, as is probably more common in addicted parents) together with the long-term consequences. One could see parallels also with Kohut's conceptualisation of how some individuals have to contend with a deeply established and global threat to the self, which can be expressed in terms of a need to attack so as to keep the upper hand (see chapter 3 in this book).

It can be assumed that a child detects not only the facts of a parent's drinking or drug-taking but also the parent's predominant attitudes towards the activity. Did Charles, for example, adopt his mother's romantic rationalisations of her drug-taking? This might seem obvious, but is an important distinction. Similarly, with, say, sexual abuse, the child has to deal not only with the assault but also with the rationalisation or threats that accompany it. These in turn can shape and add confusion to how the individual relates to their problems in later life.

*Molly*

A patient's mother had been alcohol-dependent and abused legal drugs, while her father glamorised the use of illegal drugs. During the course of treatment, Molly's internal attitude towards the drugs closely resembled those of her mother and father, perhaps a composite of the two. She saw her mother as being like an irresponsible child, who, through drink, was normally disorientated and who would, through self-neglect, induce emergency responses from others. She recalled buying drugs for her mother and using some of these herself. Molly would also sink into similar states, mobilising concern in others, and justifying the use of street drugs to seek oblivion. Her parents had spoken about the nice feeling of being 'out of it'. They conveyed an indifference towards her nascent drug use, and she acknowledged that she did not know what it was like to worry about drugs, since they had always been part of her life. There had also been drug-using partners, who had endorsed and glamorised drugs, as well as others friends who had genuinely worried about her welfare.

From my limited understanding of the transference, I think I could be seen either as a hopeful figure, trying to remove her from a desperate state of affairs, like some of her non-drug-taking friends, or as an opponent, standing in the way of the drugs and being punitive. Help was viewed suspiciously and was associated with being used or controlled. As she once remarked, 'I have always been used by others, from a little girl upwards.' Perhaps one of the difficulties in the treatment was that Molly was still acting out the role of being an adult child of drug-abusing parents and was consequently lost in the fog of her own addiction.

## Natasha

Natasha's parents had both been addicted. Having been encouraged by them to use drugs, she fought the idea that it could be a problem. Later on, however, when the problems could no longer be pushed away, relapses were followed (or were they preceded?) by a profound confusion between good and bad, a confusion that some argue is a common state of affairs in the internal world of the addict.

In cases like this, I have found value in Fairbairn's (1943) notion of the 'moral defence'. In this concept, it is argued that the child has to deal with the unwelcome fact of having had 'bad objects' (the parents), which he or she deals with by preferring to see him or herself as bad, rather than them. In this way the needed parents are spared, however innocent the child is. Fairbairn argues that 'one of his motives in becoming bad is to make his objects "good". In becoming bad he is really taking upon himself the burden of badness which appears to reside in his objects' (p. 65). During the course of Natasha's treatment, I noticed how difficult it was for her to express anger or criticism of what her parents had done, but how readily she could berate herself for being 'bad' or 'stupid'.

The next two cases are from psychotherapy assessments. Although neither presented with addictions, both patients had experienced earlier periods in which they had been afraid of becoming excessive drinkers, a fear I have found to be common at some stage in people who have lived with an alcoholic parent.

## Claire

Claire presented with bouts of depression and helpless collapse. She felt as though she slipped into a recurring sick role, with other people looking after her, contrasting with her usual sense of efficiency, if not overdrive, in areas like work. In her efficient state, she easily felt responsible for other people's problems, often to the point of trying to sort them out. There appeared a basic conflict between helplessness versus omnipotence, and a search for self-esteem through being helpful to others. Through the assessment, clues emerged of a split in the family-of-origin (and in the patient's mind) between those allied to her father (a drinker) and those allied to her mother, with her feeling caught between them. She described the impact of her father's behaviour and how the children would man the barricade on his return from drinking sessions. She felt angry at his defensiveness after sobering up and felt used by him in order to assuage his guilt. She had learned efficiency from early on, tidying up around the house and trying, it seemed, to deal with some of the emotional mess between the parents; there was some rivalry with mother who, while helping keep the family together, had adopted or endured a downtrodden, denigrated role. There seemed a useful link here to her current problems to do with not being able to depend on an encouraging object inside herself and a tendency to fall sick in response to feeling needs.

I have observed, in treating other patients, a pattern of compulsive caring having been built up, perhaps based on a real sense that an early or developing self was overburdened. With Claire, her wish to help others would escalate into a burdensome demand, from within, though consciously experienced as coming from others.

I have noticed that with some female patients, like Claire, having a baby or seeing, say, a friend or a sibling with a baby can arouse strong feelings about the past, not consciously available earlier. Burning feelings of deprivation and vulnerability can then rise to the surface.

*Gerry*

When describing his past, Gerry spoke of a large family stretched for resources. For him, this situation meant much jockeying for position, with not enough love to go round. He portrayed his father as a good man, yet too exhausted to provide a lively or strong presence, having spent his energy (in Gerry's view) on the other children. Mother's presence, by contrast, was lively but negative, due to her moods and drink problem. In fact, it was hard to know how separable the moods and the drinking were. He graphically described his early feelings of terror around his mother and the uncertainty about what kind of mother he would find, on a daily basis. He recalled having to put himself at a physical distance from her, to protect himself from the violence sometimes directed at him.

Richards (1980) comments on the way in which the wild inconsistency, the Dr Jekyll and Mr Hyde behaviour, of the drinking parent can enormously confuse and exaggerate a more normal process of splitting in the child. Similarly, although concentrating on drinking fathers, Newell (1960) talks evocatively of experiences of let-down and of a child exposed to 'a bewildering array of ambivalence, inconsistencies, antagonisms and touching overtures of affection' (p. 92).

Perhaps, for Gerry, his mother continued to represent a frightening, 'all bad' figure, while his father, who might have promised some kind of desirable contrast, proved, in Gerry's experience, to have been insufficiently strong. Gerry himself presented with disabling, black moods and feared close relationships to women, who were seen as frightening and potentially emasculating.

## Conclusions

The cases reported, with the possible exception of Sally, and countless others from clinical experience, leave little doubt about the contribution of early deprivation, confusion and damage. However, if human development is not a simple unfolding, as with Aristotle's metaphor of the acorn and the oak, nor is the concept of damage. What are the implications of this?

The AlAnon and the co-dependency movements, like ACAs, do provide an invaluable resource, a culture of acceptance to those affected by the addiction of others. At the same time, the result of parental substance misuse cannot be reduced to any particular syndrome. My own work with families and spouses affected by alcoholism, both past and current, has convinced me of the need for flexible understanding and care, not to add to the guilt that individuals usually already feel.

The case for research from ordinary community as well as clinical samples is well made by Orford and Velleman (1999). We cannot expect all negative childhood experiences to have the same, uniform, long-term effects, and resiliency needs to be understood as well as vulnerability/ susceptibility. Rutter's (1999) paper clarifies some of the implications of such views, although it does not deal specifically with addiction. He usefully reminds us of the important role of 'turning points' and 'neutralising' experiences during development and of the deleterious consequences that different 'chains of adversity' can have throughout life. A psychodynamic appreciation of such issues can be found in Bowlby's (1988b) work on developmental psychiatry and pathways.

The type of dynamic process observed in the case vignettes is not, of course, confined to individuals brought up with addiction. I have encountered, for example, the profound confusion between good and bad reported in Natasha's case in individuals exposed to childhood violence (without addiction), which acts as a constituent of later episodes of violent acting out during adolescence or adulthood. Similarly, I have seen the compulsive caring of Claire in many other patients, such as those having had an experience of mental illness or depression in a parent(s). Clinicians will readily be able to think of countless other examples.

The way the child experiences his or her parents is individual and subtle and, as Kohut (1977a) reminds us, it is not just what parents *do* that matters, but how they *are*. The overall empathic and responsive milieu of family life, or the absence of it, has to be assessed. This means the need to look beyond overt behaviour and patterns of drinking or drug use per se, and to concentrate instead on the subjective experience of the individual concerned. The same emphasis applies, in my view, to attachment theory and the potential threat to secure attachment posed by an addicted parent; we still need to understand, through the process of therapy, the individual's experience of the attachment, disruption or loss, as well as maintaining awareness of the possibility that psychic pain was mitigated through attachments to other figures in the person's life.

# References

Abraham K (1908) The psychological relations between sexuality and alcoholism. In: Selected Papers in Psychoanalysis (1979). New York: Brunner/Mazel.

Aichhorn A (1935) Wayward Youth. New York: Viking Press.

Bacal H (1995) The essence of Kohut's work and the progress of self psychology. Psychoanalytic Dialogues 5(3): 353–366.

Baker H and Baker M (1987) Heinz Kohut's self psychology: an overview. American Journal of Psychiatry 144(1): 1–9.

Ball S and Legow N (1996) Attachment theory as a working model for the therapist transitioning from early to later recovery substance abuse treatment. American Journal of Drug & Alcohol Abuse 22(4): 533–547.

Bean M and Zinberg N (eds.) (1981) Dynamic Approaches to the Understanding and Treatment of Alcoholism. New York: Free Press.

Beck AT, Wright FD, Newman CF and Liese BS (1993) Cognitive Therapy of Substance Misuse. New York: Guilford.

Beletsis S and Brown S (1981) A developmental framework for understanding the adult children of alcoholics. Journal of Addictions and Health 2: 187–203

Benedek T (1938) Adaption to reality in early infancy. Psychoanalysis Quarterly 7: 200–214.

Bion H (1967) Second Thoughts. Select Papers on Psychoanalysis. London: Heinemann Maresfield.

Bion H (1992) Cogitations. (ed. Bion F) London & New York: Karnac Books.

Bion WR (1961) Experiences in Groups and Other Papers. London: Tavistock.

Blaine J and Julius D (eds.) (1977) The Psychodynamics of Drug Dependence. NIDA Monograph, Washington DC: Government Printing Office.

Bowlby J (1979) The Making and Breaking of Affectional Bonds. London: Tavistock.

Bowlby J (1988a) A Secure Base: Parent–Child Attachment and Healthy Development. New York: Basic Books.

Bowlby J (1988b) Developmental psychiatry comes of age. American Journal of Psychiatry 145(1): 1–10.

Brown S (1997) Treating Adult Children of Alcoholics: A Developmental Perspective. Bristol: John Wiley and Sons.

Cade B and O'Hanlon WH (1993) A Brief Guide to Brief Therapy. New York: W.W. Norton.

Cermack T (1986) Diagnosing and Treating Co-dependence. Minnesota: Johnston Institute Books.

Cermack, T (1989) AlAnon and recovery. In: Galanter M (ed.) Recent Developments in Alcoholism, vol. 7. New York: Plenum Press.

Cork M (1969) The Forgotten Children: a Study of Children with Alcoholic Parents. Toronto: Addiction Research Foundation.

Cummings C, Gordon JR and Marlatt GA (1980) Relapse prevention and prediction. In: Miller WR (ed.) The Addictive Behaviours. New York: Pergamon.

De Zulueta F (1993) From Pain to Violence: The Traumatic Roots of Destructiveness. London: Whurr.

Deutsch H (1926) Occult processes occurring in psychoanalysis. In: Imago **12**: 418–433, translated from the German by George Devereux (ed.) as Psychoanalysis and the Occult (1953).

Dodes L (1990) Addiction, helplessness and narcissistic rage. Psychoanalytic Quarterly **59**: 398–416.

Edwards P, Harvey C and Whitehead P (1973) Wives of alcoholics. Quarterly Journal of Studies on Alcohol **34**: 112–132

Eissler KR (1950) Ego psychological implications of the psychoanalytic treatment of delinquents. Psychoanalytic Study of the Child **5**: 97–121.

El-Guebaly N and Offord R (1977) The offspring of alcoholics: a critical review. American Journal of Psychiatry **134**(4): 357–365

Fairbairn WRD (1943) The repression and the return of bad objects. In: Fairbairn WRD (1952) Psychoanalytic Studies of the Personality. London: Routledge and Kegan Paul.

Flowers L and Zweben J (1998) The changing role of 'using' dreams in addiction recovery. Journal of Substance Abuse Treatment **15**(3): 193–200.

Fonagy P, Moran G and Target M (1993) Aggression and the psychological self. International Journal of Psychoanalysis **74**: 41–485.

Foulkes SH (1948) Introduction to Group-analytic Psychotherapy. London: Heinemann.

Fried E (1979) Narcissistic inaccessibility. Group **3**(2): 79-87.

Freud A (1965a) The Writings of Anna Freud, vol. 6. New York: International University Press.

Freud A (1965b) Normality and Pathology in Childhood. New York: International Universities Press.

Freud S (1905) Three Essays on the Theory of Sexuality. Standard Edition of the Complete Psychological Works of Sigmund Freud, 7. London: Hogarth Press (hereafter S.E.).

Freud S (1910) The Future Prospects of Psychoanalytic Therapy. S.E. **11.**

Freud S (1912) Recommendations to Physicians Practicing Psychoanalysis. S.E. **12.**

Freud S (1913) The Disposition to Obsessional Neurosis. S.E. **12.**

Freud S (1919) Lines of Advance in Psychoanalytic Therapy. S.E. **17.**

Freud S (1923) The Ego and the Id. London: Hogarth Press.

Freud S (1928) Dostoevsky and Paricide. S.E. **21.**

Gittelson R (1952) The emotional position of the analyst in the psychoanalytic situation. International Journal of Psychoanalysis **33**: 1–10.

Glasser M (1982) Problems in the psychoanalysis of certain narcissistic disorders. International Journal of Psychoanalysis **73**: 493–503.

Glasser M (1988) Psychodynamic aspects of paedophilia. Psychoanalytic Psychotherapy **3**(2): 121–135.

Glover E (1932) On the aetiology of drug addiction. International Journal of Psycho-Analysis **13**: 298–328.

Goldberg A (1980) Advances in Self Psychology. New York: International University Press.

Gossop M (1989) Relapse and Addictive Behaviour. London: Tavistock/Routledge.

Greenson RR (1967) The Technique and Practice of Psychoanalysis. New York: International Universities Press.

Guntrip H (1969) Schizoid Phenomena. Object-relations and the Self. New York: International Universities Press.

Heard D and Lake B (1986) The attachment dynamic in adult life. British Journal of Psychiatry **149**: 430–438.

Heimann P (1949–50) On countertransference. In: Collected Papers: About Children and Children No Longer. London: The New Library of Psychoanalysis.

Heimann P (1959–1960) Countertransference. In: Collected Papers: About Children and Children No Longer. London: The New Library of Psychoanalysis.

Henry G (1974) Doubly deprived. Journal of Child Psychotherapy **4**(2): 16–29.

Hoffer W (1949) Deceiving the deceiver. In: Eissler KR (ed.) Searchlights on Delinquency 150–5. New York: Universities Press.

Hogan D (1998) Annotation. The Psychological development and welfare needs of children of opiate and cocaine users. Journal of Child Psychology and Psychiatry **5**: 609–619.

Holmes J (1993) John Bowlby and Attachment Theory. London: Routledge.

Holmes J (1996) Attachment Intimacy Autonomy: Using Attachment Theory in Adult Psychotherapy. New York: Aronson.

Hopper E (1995) A psychoanalytic theory of 'drug addiction': unconscious fantasies of homosexuality, compulsions & masturbation within the context of traumatogenic process. International Journal of Psychoanalysis **76**: 1121–1142.

Hunt W, Barnett L and Branch L (1971) Relapse rates in addiction programmes. Journal of Clinical Psychology **27**: 455–486.

Hyatt Williams A (1966) La belle dame sans merci: the bad breast mother. American Imago **63**: 63–81.

Hyatt Williams A (1978) Depression, deviation and acting out in adolescence. Journal of Adolescence **1**: 309–317.

Hyatt Williams A (1986) The Ancient Mariner: opium, the saboteur of self-therapy. Free Associations **6**: 120–144.

Imhoff J, Hirsch R and Terenzi R (1983) Countertransferential and attitudinal considerations in the treatment of drug abuse and addiction. International Journal of Addiction **18**(4): 491–510.

Kaufman E (1994) Psychotherapy of Addicted Persons. New York: Guilford Press.

Keller DS (1996) Exploration in the service of relapse prevention. In: Rotgers F, Keller D and Morgenstern J (eds.) Treating Substance Abuse: Theory and Technique. New York: Guilford Press.

Kern J (1978) Management of children of alcoholics. In: Zinberg N, Wallace J and Blum S (eds.) Practical Approaches to Alcoholism Psychotherapy. New York: Plenum Press.

Kernberg O, Seltzer M and Koenigsberg HW (1989) Psychodynamic Psychotherapy of Borderline patients. New York: Basic Books.

Khantzian EJ (1990) An ego-self theory of substance dependence. In: Lettieri DJ,

Khantzian EJ, Halliday KS and McAuliffe WE (1990) Addiction and the Vulnerable Self: Modified Dynamic Group Psychotherapy for Substance Abusers. New York: Guilford Press.

Khantzian EJ (1985) The self-medication hypothesis of addictive disorders. American Journal of Psychiatry **142**(11): 1259–1264.

Khantzian E and Treece C (1985) DSM-111 Psychiatric diagnosis of narcotic addicts. Archives of General Psychiatry **42**: 1067–1071

Khantzian EJ (1977) The self-medication of substance use disorders: a reconstruction and recent applications. Harvard Review of Psychiatry **4**(5): 231–244.

Khantzian E and Mack J (1989) Alcoholics Anonymous and contemporary psychodynamic theory. In: Galanter M (1989) Recent Developments in Alcoholism, vol. 7. New York: Plenum Press.

Klein M (1946) Notes on some schizoid mechanisms. In: Klein M et al. (1952) Developments in Psychoanalysis. London: Hogarth Press.

Klein M (1957) Envy and gratitude. In: Klein M (1984) Envy and Gratitude and Other Works. London: Hogarth Press.

Knight R (1953) Borderline states. In: Bulletin of the Menninger Clinic **17**(1): 1–12.

Kohut H (1971) The Analysis of the Self. New York: International University Press.

Kohut H (1972) Thoughts on narcissism and narcissistic rage. Psychoanalytic Study of the Child **27**: 360–400.

Kohut H (1977a) The Restoration of the Self. New York: International University Press.

Kohut H (1977b) 'Preface' of Blaine J and Julius D (1977) (see above).

Kohut H and Wolf F (1978) The disorders of the self and their treatment: an outline. International Journal of Psychoanalysis **59**: 413–426.

Krystal H (1982) Alexthymia and the effectiveness of psychoanalytic treatment. International Journal of Psychoanalytic Psychotherapy **9**: 352–378.

Laplanche J and Pontalis JB (1973) The Language of Psychoanalysis. London: Hogarth Press.

Lettieri D, Sayers M and Wallace HW (eds.) (1990) Theories of Addiction (NIDA Research Monograph No. 30, DHHS Publication No. ADM 80-967). Washington DC: US Government Printing Office.

Levin J (1987) Treatment of Alcoholism and the Addictions: A Self-psychology Approach. New York: Jason Aronson.

Limentani A (1986) On the psychodynamics of drug dependence. Free Associations **5**: 48–64.

Little M (1951) Counter-transference and the patient's response to it. In: Little M (1981) Transference Neurosis and Transference Psychosis. New York: Jason Aronson.

Mackie A (1981) Attachment theory; its relevance to the therapeutic alliance. British Journal of Medical Psychology **54**: 203–212.

Main M, Kaplan K and Cassidy J (1985) Security in infancy, childhood and adulthood. A move to the level of representation. In: Bretherton I and Waters E (eds.) Growing Points of Attachment Theory and Research. Monographs of the Society for Research in Child Development **50**: 66–104.

Mannheim J (1955) Notes on a case of drug addiction. International Journal of Psychoanalysis **36**: 66–73.

Maratos J (1988) Self psychology. Current Opinion in Psychiatry **1**: 284–288.

Marlatt A (1982) Relapse prevention: a self-control program for the treatment of addictive behaviours. In: Stuart R (ed.) Adherence, Compliance and Generalisation in Behavioural Medicine. New York: Brunner/Mazel.

Marlatt GA and Gordon JR (1980) Determinants of relapse; implications for the maintenance of behaviour change. In: Davidson P and Davidson S (eds.) Behavioural Medicine: Changing Health Lifestyles. New York: Brunner/Mazel.

Marlatt GA and Gordon JR (1985) Relapse Prevention: Maintenance Strategies in the Treatment of Addictive Behaviors. New York: Guilford.

Marrone M (1998) Attachment and Interaction. London: Jessica Kingsley Publishers.

McDougall J (1986) Theatres of the Mind. London: Free Association Books.

McDougall J (1989) Theatres of the Body. London: Free Association Books.

Miller W and Rollnick S (1991) Motivational Interviewing: Preparing People to change Addictive Behaviour. New York: Guilford Press.

Mollon P (1986) An appraisal of Kohut's contribution. British Journal of Psychotherapy 3(2): 151–161.

Moos R, Finney J and Cronkite R (1990) Alcoholism Treatment. Oxford: Oxford University Press.

Narcotics Anonymous, (1987) 4th edition. Van Nuys, California: World Service Office Inc.

Newell N (1960) Alcoholism and the father image. Quarterly Studies on Alcohol 11: 92–96.

Nyman D and Cocores J (1991) In: Miller N (ed.) Comprehensive Handbook of Drug and Alcohol Addiction. New York: Marcel Dekker Inc.

O'Neill E (1947) The Iceman Cometh. London: Jonathan Cape.

O'Neill E (1959) Long Day's Journey into Night. London: Jonathan Cape.

Obholzer A and Roberts VZ (eds.) (1994) The Unconscious at Work. London: Tavistock Publications.

Orford J (1991) Psychobiological synthesis vs. excessive appetites. Paper presented at 'The Window of Opportunity: An Intersectoral Approach to Drug-related Problems in Our Society' Conference, Adelaide, Australia, 1991.

Orford J, Daniels V and Somers M (1996) Drinking and gambling: a comparison with implications for theories of addiction. Drug and Alcohol Review 15: 47–56.

Prochaska JO, DiClemente CC and Norcross JC (1992) In search of how people change: applications to addictive behaviours. American Psychologist 47: 1102–1114.

Rado S (1933) The psychoanalysis of pharmacothymia. Psychoanalytic Quarterly 2: 1–12.

Rado S (1957) Narcotic bondage. In: Hoch P and Zubin J. (eds.) Problems of Addiction and Habituation. New York: Grune and Stratton.

Richards TM (1980) Splitting as a defence mechanism in children of alcoholics. In: Galanter M (ed.) Recent Developments in Alcoholism, vol. 7. New York: Plenum Press.

Rivinius T (1997) Children of Chemically Dependent Parents. New York: Brunner/Mazel.

Rodríguez de la Sierra L (1995) Of sentiment and sensations. British Journal of Psychotherapy 12(2).

Rogers CR (1951) Client-centred Therapy. London: Constable.

Rosenfeld H (1960) On drug addiction. In Psychotic States: A Psychoanalytic Approach. London: Hogarth Press.
Rosenfeld H (1965) The psychopathology of drug addiction and alcoholism: a critical review of the psychosomatic literature. In: Psychotic States. London: Hogarth Press.
Rutter M (1985) Resilience in the face of adversity. British Journal of Psychiatry 147: 598–611.
Rutter M (1999) Resilience concepts and findings: implications for family therapy. Journal of Family Therapy 21: 119–144.
Rycroft C (1968) A Critical Dictionary of Psychoanalysis. London: Penguin Books.
Rydelius P (1997) Annotation: are children of alcoholics a clinical concern for the child and adolescent psychiatrist of today? Journal of Child Psychology and Psychiatry 38: 615–624.
Saltzburger-Wittenberg I (1970) Psycho-analytic Insight and Relationships. London: Routledge and Kegan Paul.
Sandler J (1976) Countertransference and role responsiveness. International Review of Psychoanalysis 3: 43–47.
Schlesinger N and Robbins F (1983) A Developmental View of the Psychoanalytic Process. New York: International University Press.
Sedlack V (1989) Disavowal and assessment for psychotherapy. Psychoanalytic Psychotherapy 4(2): 97–107.
Segal H (1986) The Work of Hanna Segal. London: Free Association Books.
Spratley T (1989) A multi-disciplinary and team approach. British Journal of Addiction 84: 259–266.
Sroufe A (1979) The coherence of individual development. American Psychologist 34: 834–841.
Thompson F (1992) Collected Poems. UK: Fisher Press.
Vannicelli M (1991) Dilemmas and countertransference considerations in group psychotherapy with adult children of alcoholics. International Journal of Group Psychotherapy 41(3): 295–312.
Velleman R and Orford J (1999) Risk or Resilience: Adults Who Were the Children of Problem Drinkers. The Netherlands: Harwood Academic Publishers.
Wanigaratne SD (1997) Development and evaluation of a new model of psychology service provision for drug users. Unpublished paper, City University, London.
Wanigaratne SD, Billington A and Williams M (1997) Initiating and maintaining safer sex: evaluation of group work with gay men. In: Catalan J, Sherr L and Hedge B (eds.) The Impact of Aids: Psychological and Social Aspects of HIV Infection. Amsterdam: Harwood Academic Press.
Wanigaratne SD, Wallace W, Pullin J, Keaney F and Farmer R (1990) Relapse Prevention for Addictive Behaviours: A Manual for Therapists. Oxford: Blackwell.
Weegmann M (1993) Methadone in the Madness. Unpublished paper.
Weegmann M (2002a) (in press) Eugene O'Neill's Hughie and the grandiose addict. Psychodynamic Practice 8:1.
Weegmann M (2002b) 'Motivational interviewing and addiction: a psychodynamic appreciation'. Psychodynamic Practice 8:2.
Wegscheider S (1981) Another Chance: Hope and Health for the Alcoholic Family. Palo Alto: Science and Behaviour Books.
Weiss R (1982) Attachment in adult life. In: Parkes CM and Hinde R (eds.) The Place of Attachment in Human Behaviour. London: Routledge.

Welldon E (1993) Forensic psychotherapy and group analysis. In: Group Analysis **26**: 487–502.

Wilson C and Oford J (1978) Children of alcoholics. Journal of Studies on Alcohol **39**(1): 121–142.

Winnicott DW (1947) Further Thoughts on Babies as Persons. In Winicott (1964).

Winnicott DW (1951) Transitional objects and transitional phenomena. In: Winnicott (1951) Collected Papers: Through Paediatrics to Psychoanalysis. London: Tavistock.

Winnicott DW (1964) The Child, the Family and the Outside World. London: Penguin Books.

Woody GE, Luborsky L and McLellan AT (1983) Psychotherapy for opiate addicts. Archives of General Psychiatry **40**: 639–645.

Woody GE, McLellan AT and Luborsky L (1995) Psychotherapy in community methadone programs: a validation study. American Journal of Psychiatry **152**: 1302–1308.

Wurmser L (1978) The Hidden Dimension: The Psychopathology of Compulsive Drug Use. New York: Jason Aronson.

Yorke C (1970) A critical review of some psychoanalytic literature on drug addiction. British Journal of Medical Psychology **43**: 151–184.

Zinberg N (1975) Addiction and ego function. Psychoanalytic Study of the Child **30**: 567–588.

Zoja L (1989) Drugs, Addiction and Ritual. Boston: Sigo Press.

# Index

177